ALKALINE HERBAL MEDICINE

Reverse Disease and
Heal the Electric Body

CONTENTS

CHAPTER 1: MEDICINAL HERBS—SUPPORTING THE ELECTRIC AFRICAN GENOME ECOSYSTEM

Plants and the Ecosystem WHAT IS A MEDICINAL HERB?
Medicinal Herbs and the Body's Natural Healing Process MEDICINAL HERBS FOR THE ELECTRIC GENOME OF *HOMO SAPIENS* The Electric African Genome and Body Neanderthal Genome
Healthy Expression of the Common African Genome CHAPTER 2: ALKALINE PLANT FOOD ALKALINE PLANT FOODS AND HERBS SUPPORT THE ALKALINE BODY WATER

PROTEIN?

Nitrogen Saturated Plant Foods MILK

ENERGY

CLEANSING

OILS

SEASONINGS

HERBAL TEAS

SUGARS

CHAPTER 3: PREPARING HERBS HARVESTING MEDICINAL HERBS Roots

Leaves
Flowers
Drying Herbs

BULK HERBS

MAKING HERBS

INFUSION

Preparation

DECOCTION

Preparation

GRINDING HERBS, ENCAPSULATION, AND DOSAGE Grinding

Encapsulation
Dosage

CHILDREN'S DOSAGES

Clarke's Rule

CHAPTER 4: ALKALINE MEDICINAL HERBS HERBS AND THEIR PROPERTIES Arnica

- Batana
- Bladderwrack
- Blessed Thistle
- Blue Vervain
- Burdock Root
- Cascara Sagrada
- Chaparral
- Cocolmeca
- Contribo
- Damiana
- Elderberry
- Eyebright
- Guaco
- Huereque
- Hombre Grande
- Hops
- Hydrangea
- Lavender
- Lily of the Valley
- Nettle
- Nopal
- Prodigiosa
- Red Clover
- Rhubarb Root
- Sage
- Santa Maria
- Sapo
- Sarsaparilla
- Sea Moss
- Sensitiva
- Shea Butter
- Tila
- Urtila Oil
- Valerian
- Yellow Dock
- Yohimbe

OLD SEBI HERBS
- Current Estro Product
- Past Estro Product

OTHER-SEBI HERBS
- Guinea Hen Weed
- Mullein

NON-SEBI HERBS
- Black Seed

CHAPTER 5: HERBAL COMBINATIONS DR. SEBI'S HERBAL PRODUCTS Cell

Products
>	Packages
COMBINING HERBS
>	Parts
>	The Foundation
>	Calcification Remover
>
>	Pancreas and Endocrine Support Gut and Cell Cleanser
>
>	Brain and Nerve Support Uterine Support (Antifibroid) Vaginal Canal Wash
>	Male Support
>	Cell Energizer
>	Nutrient Support
>	Lupus Buster
>	Complex Diseases

CHAPTER 6: RESOURCES DR. SEBI'S OFFICE, INC.
HERBS OF MEXICO
NATURAL LIFE ENERGY
THE GOD AWAKENING DIET ABOUT THE AUTHOR

NOTES

CHAPTER 1:

MEDICINAL HERBS—SUPPORTING THE ELECTRIC AFRICAN GENOME

We live in an amazing ecosystem that is responsible for supporting all life. When we think of life, we often think of the big things we see like people, animals, trees, and plants. Life is much more than that and is made up greatly of organisms we normally don't see. Abundant microorganisms are responsible for keeping the bigger picture going. There is a natural balance of what we call "good" or "bad" microorganisms present all around us.

The bigger things in life, like people and animals, develop out of reactions to this balance of smaller things, or "good" and "bad" bacteria. This microbial balance is determined by the intelligent order within the earth's ecosystem and the universe that extends to our bodies, and it balances positive and negative, or primal opposites, down to the atomic level and below. I have termed this intelligent order God/the Source/Nature in an attempt to encompass all views that recognize this order in one way or another.

This intelligent order that produces the balance of positive and negative, or push and pull, produces energy that is responsible for the various forces within the ecosystem and in all life. In the body, the healthy state of energy is supported by the consumption of a specific combination and ratio of nutrients needed to support the metabolic processes of organs, which is predetermined by the African genome. The African genome has been determined to be the foundational genome of all *Homo sapiens* or modern people. The healthy expression of the African genome present in all people is achieved in a specific way, which is predetermined by God/the Source/Nature , and a good way to better understand this process is to better understand how an ecosystem works.

ECOSYSTEM

My eye-opening experience into the workings of an ecosystem and its complex and predetermined order was a result of having fish tank. You may think that it is a simple thing to maintain a healthy environment in a fish tank, but it is not so easy. There needs to be a natural balance that has been intelligently determined. I soon realized I needed to mimic the natural balance that exists in fresh and saltwater sources in nature to provide a healthy environment for the fish in the tank.

    I thought maintaining a fish tank would be as easy as adding some water, some rocks, and some fish, and feeding them. This wasn't the case, and in a very short time, the water became murky with dissolved fish feces and harmful bacteria. I learned the hard way that if the environment didn't closely mimic the fish's natural environment, I would not be able to maintain a healthy fish tank. The environment needed for the fish to survive and thrive is predetermined. I learned that everything in the tank interacted with each other, from the microorganisms, to the minerals, to the food, to the pH level of the water, to its oxygen level, and a specific balance was needed.

    I had to remove synthetic chemicals that were added to the tap water I used to fill the fish tank. Chemicals like chlorine quickly attacked the health of the fish. I needed to add good bacteria to the water and have a place for it to grow so it could feed on the compounds in the fish's feces and produce byproducts like oxygen to keep the water healthy. The good bacteria counteracted the growth of the bad bacteria by cutting off its food supply. The good bacteria also kept the nutrients in balance, which supported the desired pH and oxygen level in the tank. I feel that the most important thing I did to support the overall health of the tank and the fish was adding plants. Plants play a very important role in maintaining life in the earth's ecosystem, and this includes not only the health of life on land but also the health of life in oceans, lakes, and streams, and in this case, the fish tank.

Plants and the Ecosystem

Plant life played a very important role in maintaining the health of the fish tank and fish, and it plays an equally important role in the earth's ecosystem. Like plants that grow on land through the absorption of minerals in the soil, plants in the tank absorbed nitrates and other compounds in the fish poop to grow. Plants in both environments convert carbon dioxide (CO_2) produced by animals into oxygen (O_2), which animals need to carry out metabolic processes. Plants on land clean the air, and plants in natural water sources and in the tank clean the water, which serves to protect life in both environments. Plants also serve as a food source, and their nutrient makeup bolsters the immune systems of animals.

The unhealthy environment in the tank was a result of going against the predetermined or intelligent order, which brought about unbalance and the proliferation of disease. When I put plants into this environment, they generally were able to resist disease, rebalance the nutrients in the water, and create an environment that was inhospitable to disease.

I observed that the plants in the tank were much hardier than the fish in the face of unbalance. Their hardiness helped them survive in unfavorable conditions and gave them the time to put the environment in the fish tank back into balance. The plants' nutrient composition and specifically their phytonutrient makeup helped protect them against the unbalance and unhealthy environment in the tank. The fish would feed on the plants and consume their nutrients and phytonutrients, which would strengthen the fish's immune system and offer added defense against the inhospitable environment.

The consumption of plant life is necessary for the continued survival of animals on land as well as fish in the sea, directly or indirectly. Directly, some animals primarily or totally survive by eating plants to get their predetermined and required amounts of nutrients (vitamins, minerals, carbohydrates, protein, and fat) to support metabolic processes and phytonutrients (carotenoids and flavonoids, for example) to help support their immune system. Indirectly, other animals primarily or totally survive by eating animals that graze on plants to get their nutrients and phytonutrients. So consuming plant life is the root of supporting health.

The consumption of plants is supportive of health because of the nutrients and phytonutrients they contain. Different plants and the fruit they bear contain different concentrations and varieties of nutrients and phytonutrients. Observing reactions to the consumption of plants and their fruit led to the development of traditional practices using them to combat disease and to support health. In general, all natural plants offer some level of healing and maintenance of health. Some plants have a stronger concentration of nutrients and phytonutrients, and these plants usually serve as herbal medicines to reverse disease, rather than as food to be consumed in large amounts on a daily basis. Usually these herbs are bitter and don't make for the best dishes, and they can have side effects if taken in large doses or for too long.

WHAT IS A MEDICINAL HERB?

Before the invention of allopathic or Western pharmacological medicine, people were actually able to reverse disease using natural or traditional medicine made from plants. The Western paradigm, corporate structure, and medical institutions would like you to think otherwise. Around 50 percent of pharmaceutical drugs made during the last thirty years were made either directly or indirectly from plants.[1] Before the globalization of the world into a socioeconomic system that marginalized the poor in so-called third-world countries and conditioned people to only have faith in Western pharmacological medicine, indigenous people all around the world were more in tune with the environment and understood which plants to consume to reverse disease. Plant herbs were recognized for their healing properties going all the way back to Dynastic Egypt and before.

All plants contain nutrients and phytonutrients and provide some level of health-enhancing properties. Medicinal herbs and food herbs or food spices differ from plant foods due to their higher concentration of nutrients and phytonutrients, which result in either a highly bitter taste or a highly aromatic or pungent taste. Medicinal herbs like cardo santo or hombre grande are primarily derived from flowers, roots, and barks and are bitterer and usually more potent in reversing disease than food herbs. Food herbs like rosemary and thyme are primarily derived from plant leaves, and small amounts of these spices add highly aromatic or pungent flavors to food. Because of their higher concentration of nutrients and phytonutrients, these herbs are sometimes used in higher dosages and serve as medicinal herbs in traditional medicine.

Medicinal Herbs and the Body's Natural Healing Process

The body is a wonderful and complex machine that was designed to self-correct. It was designed to resist and kill disease, repair damaged cells, and if necessary, destroy severely damaged cells. Within the life span of a person, the body is constantly working to replace old cells with new cells by replicating cells. This is how the body maintains the overall health of its blood and organs. Most cells in the body replace themselves and die off in a programmed process called apoptosis.[2][3][4] Red blood cells replace themselves around every four months, bones around every ten years, the lining of the stomach and intestines around every five days, and skin around every two to four weeks. Brain cells weren't thought to regenerate, but now science is reevaluating this idea.[5] The body carries out these processes using hormones and proteins. Phytonutrients assist these molecules in their jobs and maintain the health of the organs that produce them. This design is so complex it could only have been created by an intelligent order.

When people consume plants and their phytonutrients, their bodies are able to use the organic compounds to bolster the immune system. These phytonutrients can kill cancer cells, help repair DNA, detoxify and bind with toxins so they can be removed from the body, enhance cell communication, kill pathogens, and serve as antioxidants to protect cells from free radical damage and aging. Phytonutrients are divided into classes, including carotenoids, flavonoids, phytates, ligans, isothiocyanates or indoles, phenols, saponins, sulfides, and terpenes, and they all interact with the body in various ways.

When it is time for cells to replicate, the body does all it can to make sure the cells that are being replicated are healthy. It will use its own internal processes and will also use nutrients and phytonutrients it gets from plants to ensure cells are replicated without any damage from pathogens or toxins. Specific phytonutrients can interact with predetermined cells, pathogens, and toxins to clean those cells and neutralize the pathogens and toxins. Phytonutrients like the flavonoids in the elderberry herb can bind with the H1N1 flu virus and block it from entering cells, while phytonutrients from other plants are not able to do the same. Phytonutrients from some plants are recognized by cell receptors and are able to enter various cells and clean the cells of pathogens and toxins, while others are limited to neutralizing pathogens and toxins in the bloodstream. Herbs like cardo santo and cascara sagrada are used to clean cells on the intracellular level.

MEDICINAL HERBS FOR THE ELECTRIC GENOME OF *HOMO SAPIENS*

The African body is the archetype of human development. Human life began in Africa and then spread to different parts of the world. Whether you believe solely in evolution or religion or a combination of the two, careful and unbiased analysis will lead you to Africa for the start of the human journey. Africa is responsible for the modern human lineage throughout the world. Navigating through the obstacles of racism, prejudice, and political and economic agendas, evolutionary science has finally been able to acknowledge that modern human life came out of Africa and spread throughout the world.

The Electric African Genome and Body

The environment in Africa fully supported the African genome, and the African genome is the foundation for all human life. The environment included the way the sun affected the development of life, the air and balance of elements in it, and the minerals and compounds in the soil. Microorganisms, plant life, animal life, and human life developed in specific ways directly out of their interaction with the ecosystem in Africa. Take something out, and life develops differently. Add something, and life develops differently. The interaction of the Africans and the African ecosystem developed a body that was highly electric and alkaline. This supported optimal physical and mental well-being and put the Africans in tune with the healing environment of the African ecosystem.

    The African body has a predetermined state of homeostasis that is determined through its genetics. Homeostasis is the state where all of the body's organs operate at their optimal level. Either this genetic structure developed out of a reaction to the ecosystem of Africa, or the genetic structure was programmed by an intelligent order I refer to as God/the Source/Nature . I coined the term God/the Source/Nature in an attempt to encompass all views that recognize this order in life in one way or another.

    The environmental factors of Africa and the general lifestyle supported the predetermined state of homeostasis in the body. The plant-centered diets of the early Africans, which emphasized the consumption of alkaline plants, naturally supported the electrical balance and healthy expression of the African genome. Looking at this subject from a scientific perspective, African humans were supposed to have evolved from the great apes, which were primarily plant eaters. The great apes were predisposed or predetermined through their genetics to consume primarily plant foods. A natural evolution would also predispose humans to primarily eat plants to support the healthy expression of their genetic structure. The environment of Africa, with its predominantly warm climate, supported the growth of plant food year-round. The reliance on the consumption of meat was introduced by Neanderthals, which were forced to adapt to their less hospitable environment. This came at a price of the unhealthy expression of the African genome, the expression of disease, and the mutation of the African genome.

The plant life that grew in Africa grew within the same environmental conditions as the Africa body. It developed with a wider range of nutrients and a complete structure that had chemical affinity with African genome. These plants were digested without producing byproducts that harmed the body or threw it out of homeostasis. The natural plant foods and herbs fully supported the healthy expression of the African genome. These natural plant foods were highly alkaline in nature and contained an optimal balance of carbohydrates, fats, proteins, vitamins, and minerals that supported a highly electrical state in the body, which promoted optimal physical, mental, and emotional well-being.

Natural plants that grew outside Africa, like flowers used as medicinal herbs, also provided support for the African genome. They may have been more resilient in some aspects because they had to develop their phytonutrients to withstand harsher environmental conditions. The coldness and reduced sun of the environment didn't support year-round growth of medicinal herbs.

Natural plants are plants that haven't been hybridized through human intervention. Many of the plants eaten today are the result of man-made hybridization of two or more plants. This negatively affects the natural balance of nutrients in plants and results in plants that are more acidic and that negatively affect the state of homeostasis and electrical activity in the body.

This state of homeostasis predetermined by the African genome was highly electrical, and the consumption of natural plant foods supplied the nutrients in the ratio needed to optimally support the quickest transmission of energy throughout the body. The body can be looked at as one big battery, and eating a diet centered on natural plants keeps the battery optimally charged. Just like a battery, using the body reduces its strength or electrical charge. Luckily the body is like a rechargeable battery, and when natural plants are consumed, nutrients in the correct ratio are added back to recharge the body.

All the functions in our bodies, such as thinking, contracting muscles, and moving fluids, are controlled by electrical signals transmitted through the nervous system. The nervous system is a two-way system that allows electrical signals to be sent back and forth from the brain and every organ in the body. These signals jump from cell to cell until the messages reach their destination, and these messages are delivered almost instantaneously under normal circumstances. The body is able to generate this electricity through the interaction of electrolytes.

Electrolytes are compounds that become ions and take on either a positive or a negative charge when they interact with water in the body. This results in positively charged ions (cations) such as calcium, magnesium, potassium, or sodium, and negatively charged ions (anions) like chloride or phosphorous. The movement and interaction of the positive and negative electrolytes across cell membranes results in the generation of electricity. Electrolytes keep the heart pumping, allow metabolic processes to happen within cells, allow organs to function properly, and allow muscles to work.

Electrolytes are needed in a specific and predetermined ratio to optimally support the health and vitality of the body, and the kidneys are constantly at work to maintain the predetermined ratio of electrolytes in the blood. A major impedance to the optimal flow of electricity in the body is excess fat. Electricity travels quicker through water than through fat, and excess fat in the body interferes with electricity's ability to quickly deliver impulses to where they are needed. The consumption of diets centered on whole plant foods supply fat in the diet at around 10 percent of the calories eaten. This percentage naturally provides the best ratio of fat to support metabolic processes, and it supports the unimpeded delivery of electrical messages throughout the body.

Not only do natural plant foods supply electrolytes and nutrients that are more supportive of the healthy expression of the African genome, but also their composition leans toward the alkaline side of the pH scale. This was perfect for keeping the blood slightly alkaline, because the body works to maintain a pH level in the blood around 7.4. Feeding the body too much acidic foods, which includes meat, dairy, and processed foods, causes the body to leech alkaline material from other areas of the body, like bones, to put them into the bloodstream to keep it slightly alkaline. An alkaline environment in the blood supported proper oxygenation of cells and metabolic processes. This also supported a healthy immune system to seek and destroy pathogens and toxins. Africa naturally produced plants that fed the African genome nutrients in the proper amount and combinations to support optimal electrical activity and oxygenation of the body, which resulted in a highly energetic, healthy, vibrant, mind and body.

Neanderthal Genome

The latest evolutionary model identified Africans in Africa as true *Homo sapiens*. Neanderthals are believed to have shared a common ancestor with African *Homo sapiens*, but they had a slightly different genome or genetic makeup. Genetic scientists have been able to isolate genetic information that is specific to Neanderthals and to Denisovans that does not exist in Africans, who did not intermix with them.[6]

A current and widely accepted scientific model supports the theory that African *Homo sapiens*, Neanderthals, and Denisovans shared a common ancestor and developed along three different lines. Another theory is the ancient human *Homo heidelbergensis* inhabited Africa and a group left Africa two to three hundred thousand years ago and then split again. The Africans who remained in Africa became *Homo sapiens*. The group that left Africa mutated to become Neanderthals and inhabited the caves of the Neandertal, also called the Neander Valley, which is a small river valley in Germany. The Neanderthals who later split from their group moved eastward into Asia and mutated again to become the lesser known Denisovan hominid. It is more likely that Neanderthals and Denisovans developed out of a mutation of the African genome, rather than all three being a mutation of a common ancestor.

Neanderthal and Denisovan DNA contains the African genome plus other genetic information. If Neanderthals and Denisovans shared a common ancestor with *Homo sapiens*, then the *Homo sapiens* genome should contain different information from those of Neanderthals and Denisovans. It appears the African *Homo sapiens* genome is the common factor, while additional information in the genome produced the Neanderthals and Denisovans.

Science indicates that the Neanderthal and Denisovan genomes were found outside of Africa, which points to these genomes developing outside of Africa. It is likely that the environmental conditions outside of Africa influenced a different expression of the African genome over hundreds of thousands of years.

The African genome was influenced or was expressed differently through its interaction with the European and East Asian environments over hundreds of thousands of years. This is likely the reason for the development of the

Neanderthal and Denisovan genomes. The less hospitable environment had a significant impact on the expression of the African genome and likely modified it.

For instance, Africans in Africa generally lived in a very warm and sunny climate. The skin of Africans contained a lot of melanin to protect them from the UV radiation of the sun. This either developed through evolution or existed through intelligent design. Since Africans normally spent a lot of time in the sun, more melanin was needed, which resulted in more protection. The melanin regulated the absorption of UV rays, which resulted in the slower production of vitamin D in the blood throughout the day.

Since Neanderthals lived in colder climates, their bodies developed proteins to toughen their skins to better deal with the cold climate. They also lost melanin and protection against UV rays. This enabled them to produce vitamin D at a quicker rate when exposed the sun. Their offspring inherited these differences through their passed-down genes, which goes to support the point that the environment can change genes and the way they are expressed. There are differences between the African *Homo sapiens* genome and the Neanderthal genome, and it is important to understand how the differences could manifest themselves.

The genetic scientists and authors of the Neanderthal ancestry study[7] found genetic variants associated with Neanderthals that affect "lupus, biliary cirrhosis, Crohn's disease, optic-disk size and type 2 diabetes and also some behaviors, such as the ability to stop smoking." The interaction of the African body with the European environment over hundreds of thousands of years led to the expression of the genome that introduced susceptibility to various diseases.

The Neanderthals lived in caves in the Neander Valley and ate diets that were heavily centered on meat consumption, because their environment wasn't supportive of the growth of lush and varied vegetation year-round. The plant life that did grow in Europe's less hospitable environment had to contend with a much colder environment and nutrient-deficient soil, compared to the more hospitable environment of Africa and similar environments like the Caribbean and Central and South America. The lifestyle and the environment of the Neanderthals did not sufficiently support the healthy expression of the African genome, resulting in an expression that promoted the development of disease.

Africans started another migration out of Africa around thirty thousand years ago. During this migration, Africans settled and built communities among themselves in different areas outside of Africa, but they also crossed the paths of

Neanderthals and Denisovans. Neanderthals and Denisovans don't exist today, and it was hypothesized that the process of natural selection produced infertility in Neanderthals and Denisovans that led to their extinction. DNA analysis paints another picture of Africans interbreeding with Neanderthals and Denisovans, producing hybrid African/Neanderthal and African/Denisovan people of Europe and Eastern Asia.

The common aspect of the genomes of the African, African/Neanderthal, and African/Denisovan peoples is the African genome. As the Africans intermixed with the African/Neanderthals and African/Denisovans, the reintroduction of the complete African genome helped stabilize the mutation done to the genome and helped support a healthier expression of the African genome in the African/Neanderthals and African/Denisovans. The African genome needs to be fully expressed to develop a highly electric and healthy body, and this is done by feeding it a diet centered on the consumption of natural plant foods and herbs that have chemical affinities with the African genome.

Diets centered on the consumption of meat, along with environmental conditions, likely led to the mutation of the African genome over hundreds of thousands of years and to the development of the Neanderthal and Denisovan genomes, which have markers for various diseases.

Healthy Expression of the Common African Genome

In order to support the complete and healthy expression of the African genome, which is the foundation for all human life, and not the expression of disease that is associated with conditions that produced the Neanderthal, is it necessary to at least return to the consumption of a plant-centered diet. Plant-centered diets are diets that consist mostly but not entirely of plant foods. Occasionally people ate meat as part of a plant-centered diet, but its consumption played a minimal part in the diet. Plant-centered diets were the norm in Africa and other places in the world that shared similar environments, like Central and South America, the Caribbean, and India, and these diets better promoted the healthy expression of the African genome. Moving away from this diet as the Neanderthals did led to the unhealthy expression of the African genome and disease.

Consuming a plant-based diet, a diet composed entirely of plant foods, is more effective than consuming a plant-centered diet for the healthiest expression of the African genome. A plant-based diet and plant herbs are vitally important when attempting to reverse disease, because they greatly limit the amount of toxins and unhealthy compounds derived from meat that enter the body and undermine the healthy expression of the African genome. It is hardwired in the African genome that the consumption of plants promotes the healthy expression of the genome, which results in physical, mental, and emotional stability. The harsher conditions of the European environment and a diet that centered on meat consumption led to the expression of the Neanderthal genome and the diseases associated with it.

Not only is the consumption of plants necessary for the healthy expression of the genome, but natural plants most effectively support the genome because they have chemical affinities with it. The genome programs the body to effectively assimilate natural plants because their chemical structure supports the expression of the genome without the development of disease in the body. The hospitable environment of Africa and environments similar to Africa, with its nutrient-dense soil, nurturing weather, and ample life-sustaining sunshine, allowed for the development of the African genome that was complete and healthy. The same environment allowed for the natural development of plant life that had complete structures and genetic profiles that had chemical affinities with the African genome and supported health instead of disease.

Plants supported the health of the body in two ways. One, they provided a wide array of minerals, vitamins, carbohydrates, fats, and protein in ratios that naturally supported the ratio of nutrients in the body. The body was able to use the nutrients to replace the nutrients lost through metabolic processes that support organ function. Two, the body was able to use plant's phytonutrients, specific and varied chemical compounds in plants, which the plants used to protect themselves against disease. The hospitable environment of Africa and similar environments abundantly and naturally produced plants that amply supplied both.

Some plants do grow in less hospitable environments outside of Africa that may or may not be an overall good source of a wide range of nutrients. They do often contain phytonutrients that protect against various diseases. Some plants can be very resilient and are able to survive in very harsh conditions through the use of their phytonutrients, and we often look to these plants for their medicinal properties. These plants are often referred to as weeds, because of their ability to find ways to grow even when their growth is not wanted. The natural plants in both hospitable and inhospitable environments support the health of the body.

The unnatural hybridization of plants lessens the chemical affinity they have with the African genome, and these plants promote the development of disease instead of supporting homeostasis and optimal functioning of all the organs and metabolic processes in the body. Multiple hybridizations severely increase the chance of the development of compounds that don't have chemical affinities with the body, even though the hybridized plants maintain some nutritional value. We have to focus on the consumption of natural plants, whether as food or as herbs, to fully support the healthy expression of the African genome, which is the root for health in all people.

All people, Africans and all descendants of Africans, should focus on the consumption of plant-centered diets and even plant-based diets based on eating natural nonhybrid plants to optimally support physical, mental, and emotional well-being. Africans have been assimilated into eating foods that are foreign to their African genome through slavery, colonialism, and globalization. It is evident that the Western diet promotes the development of chronic disease, disease that is also associated with the Neanderthal genome. European history has been riddled with chronic disease in comparison to Africa and similar countries before colonialism and slavery. The same meat-centered diet that led to the breakdown or unhealthy expression of the African genome and development of the Neanderthal genome is being globalized, with the addition of unnaturally hybridized plants and processed foods.

Put simply, health is attained through the removal of the consumption of these foods, while saturating the body with natural plants and their nutrients that were provided by God/the Source/Nature . These plants have chemical affinities with the body and support the reversal of disease and the healthy expression of the African genome. Science has recognized that some people may have a genetic disposition that puts them at risk for a certain disease, but science also supports that environmental factors like the foods you eat play a greater role in determining the expression of the genes and the risk of developing chronic disease.

The differences between the environments in Africa, Europe, and East Asia led animals and plants to develop differently. The abundance of natural resources in Africa and its ample sunshine encouraged the development of life that was vibrant and literally full of energy or electricity. The interaction of the sun and abundance of natural elements in the environment stimulated the development of life that was saturated with those elements or minerals, which promoted mental and physical vibrancy.

CHAPTER 2:

ALKALINE PLANT FOOD

We need to change the Western diet, which is being globalized, from being centered on meat, dairy, processed foods, and hybridized and genetically modified plant foods, to a diet that is centered on the consumption of alkaline plant foods. We must look to the plant foods that are indigenous to Africa or other areas of the world that share the same or similar environmental conditions of Africa, like Central and South America, the Caribbean, and India. These foods grow under the same conditions that supported and developed the African genome and supported and developed the genome of the plants that have chemical affinities with the African genome, which is the foundation of the human genome in all people.

Healing starts with removing foods that introduce toxins and pathogens and that acidify the body, cause mucus buildup, cause chronic inflammation, and lead to the development of chronic disease. The World Health Organization (WHO) released a report classifying the consumption of processed meat as "carcinogenic to humans" and the consumption of red meat as "probably carcinogenic to humans."[8] Countless scientific studies support the assertion that animal protein and animal fat increase the risk of cancer, heart disease, diabetes, and other chronic diseases.

To support the healing process and homeostasis of all the organs and functions in the body, we need to return to a diet centered on the consumption of nonhybrid whole plant foods. This is the foundation for health and healing. To speed healing or to reverse complex diseases, we should also return to using natural alkaline nonhybrid plant herbs.

The herbalist Dr. Sebi was pivotal in reestablishing the idea that alkaline nonhybrid plant foods had chemical affinities with the body and supported healing. His African Bio Mineral Balance methodology of healing is based on the premise that food that raises the acidity level in the body and that causes the overproduction of mucus in the body is the root of disease. Basically, acidic and toxin-laden foods continuously attack the body, cause a prolonged inflammatory reaction, and lead to chronic inflammation.

Acute inflammation is a natural and health-supporting process used to fight infection and to repair physical damage done to the body. When acute inflammation is not turned off, the process then attacks healthy cells in various areas of the body and leads to the development of various forms of disease. This compromises the protective mucous membrane that lines the organs and promotes excess mucus production, which in turn compromises the health of organs. So we start with removing these foods from the diet, which include meat, dairy, processed foods, and unnatural acidic hybrid plant foods. A good place to start is with this list of foods based on the alkaline foods recommended by Dr. Sebi.[9]

ALKALINE PLANT FOODS AND HERBS SUPPORT THE ALKALINE BODY

The body succumbs to disease when it is acidified. Acidifying the body compromises the mucous membrane that protects organs, which leads to the development of chronic disease. Though the different areas of the body have various pH levels, we need to consume alkaline foods that maintain the 7.4 pH (a range between 7.35 and 7.45) that the body maintains in the blood.

The term *pH* stands for "potential hydrogen" and is the ability of molecules to attract hydrogen ions. The higher the pH the lower the amount of hydrogen is available. The lower the pH the higher the amount of hydrogen is available. The scale for pH ranges from 0 to 14. The value 0 represents the highest acidic level, 7 is neutral, and 14 represents the highest alkaline level.

Stomach: Has a pH of 1.35 to 3.5, but the "mucous neck cells" that are right below the surface of the stomach lining have a neutral pH.[10]

Skin: The outer layer has a pH around 4.0 to protect it from the bacteria in the environment, and the inner layer has a pH around 6.9.[11]

Vagina: Has a pH around 4.5 to protect against microbial overgrowth.[12]

Pancreas: Has a pH between 8.0 and 8.3.

Intestines: The small intestine has a pH range of 6.0–7.4, and the large intestine has a pH range of 5.7–6.7.[13]

Blood: Has a pH range between 7.35 and 7.45.

Even though different parts of the body have different pH levels, the blood is the point of equilibrium for homeostasis in the body. Homeostasis is the tendency toward a relatively stable equilibrium between interdependent elements. The body works diligently to maintain this stable equilibrium by delivering the nutrients that organs need to maintain health.

The blood needs to maintain a 7.4 pH before it can try to maintain homeostasis in the body. Metabolic acidosis occurs when the blood's pH drops below this level, which can result in shock and death. It is important to maintain this slightly alkaline state in the blood, because it reduces the amount of hydrogen in the blood. Too much hydrogen in the blood contributes to the reduction of hemoglobin in red blood cells, which impairs the proper delivery of oxygen and nutrients to cells throughout the body. This compromises the health of the organs and metabolic functions.

The body has buffering systems in place that maintain the 7.4 pH. The buffering systems become overtaxed when the body is constantly fed acidic foods. The body will then strip alkaline material like calcium from bones and from fluids throughout the body to put into the blood to maintain its pH. This compromises the health of organs and their metabolic functions and leads to the development of chronic diseases like osteoporosis,[14] kidney disease, heart disease, and liver disease. Alkaline plant foods and herbs maintain the blood's pH without the body having to compensate and compromise its health.

WATER

Water is often overlooked but is vitally important for supporting the healthy expression of the human genome. Fruits and vegetables contain a high concentration of water, but people who consume a Western diet don't consume enough fruits and vegetables. Generally, we should consume one gallon of water a day, including water in food as well as drinking water. The safe bet would be to drink a gallon of water, and the body will get rid of what it doesn't need. Spring water is the safer water to drink. It contains natural minerals that buffer the water and protect against harmful bacteria. Drinking tap water should be avoided. Tap water contains added chemicals like chlorine to kill bacteria and fluoride to protect teeth, but these chemicals are toxic to the body and undermine homeostasis.

PROTEIN?

Dr. Sebi didn't promote the term or concept of protein because it interfered with his approach to healing. He focused on minerals or elements instead. Elements like nitrogen are the building blocks of muscle and enzymes. Nitrogen based structures in the body, like muscles and enzymes, are supported through the assimilation of nitrogen compounds. People have been conditioned to think they need to get these nitrogen compounds by consuming meat and this is not true. Plants contain nitrogen based compounds like meat, which are referred to as proteins. These nitrogenous organic compounds consist of large molecules of amino acids that are components of muscle, hair, collagen, enzymes, and antibodies.

Since a study done in 1914 showed infant rats grew faster consuming animal protein rather than vegetable protein,[15] a potent campaign had been run by the meat industry to keep animal protein as the king of protein. The campaign was so successful that many people don't realize plants contain protein and think it is necessary to consume meat to get these nitrogen compounds. This campaign was and is still used to promote the consumption of a Western diet, which is strongly tied to the development of chronic diseases. Besides the campaign's success in making some people forget that plants contain protein, it was also successful in making many people think that plant protein was an incomplete protein. This meant that plant protein didn't contain the nine essential amino acids that the body doesn't produce and that must be consumed.

The 1914 study's conclusion that vegetable protein was an incomplete protein was proved incorrect, but it didn't matter much. The meat industry was able to influence health organizations to promote the consumption of meat protein over vegetable sources of nitrogen compounds, and it was etched in the minds of the general population that the consumption of meat protein was necessary for optimal growth and health. Proponents of a plant-based diet and plant-based protein like John McDougall, MD,[16] were able to keep the pressure on these health organizations. Organizations like the American Heart Association had to finally acknowledge that plant protein was a complete protein, and protein combining wasn't necessary to achieve the daily recommended value for protein. The organization only recently released this statement on their website: "Whole grains, legumes, vegetables, seeds and nuts all contain both essential and non-essential amino acids. You don't need to consciously combine these foods ('complimentary proteins') within a given meal."[17] This information is now available on the website, but many people aren't aware of the statement and continue to think vegetable protein is an inferior protein.

Animal protein was labeled as the superior protein because infant rats grew faster while consuming it. There was also a drawback to this growth, which was not publicized or focused on. The composition or ratio of the amino acids in meat protein more closely resembled the makeup of the amino acids in the body, which is why its consumption supported accelerated growth. It also supported accelerated growth of cancer cells when consumed as more than 10 percent of the daily calories.[18] The same association was not found with the consumption of vegetable protein. The composition of vegetable protein regulates growth to naturally support human growth without supporting the growth of harmful organisms or undermining the health of cells.

Nitrogen Saturated Plant Foods

Though all plants contain complete amino acids, certain plant foods contain a higher concentration of nitrogen compounds than others. Grains, legumes, nuts, and seeds generally contain more protein than fruits and vegetables.

Grains: Amaranth, fonio, kamut, quinoa, rye, spelt, teff, wild rice **Legumes:** Garbanzo beans (chickpeas) **Nuts and seeds:** Brazil nuts, hemp seeds, pine nuts, raw sesame "tahini" butter, walnuts

MILK

Hemp-seed milk, coconut milk, walnut milk. (It is better to make your own milk than to buy it to make sure you are drinking pure nut or seed milk. See recipes.)

ENERGY

Fruits are concentrated with natural carbohydrates and are the body's natural and primary source of energy. It is better to consume fresh fruits and not canned fruits, which are processed and can contain cancer-causing additives and preservatives.

Apples, bananas, berries, cantaloupe, cherries, currants, dates, figs, grapes (seeded), key limes, mango, melons (seeded), oranges, papayas, peaches, pears, plums, prickly pear, prunes, raisins (seeded), soft jelly coconuts, soursops, tamarind

CLEANSING

Vegetables are high in micronutrients including vitamins, minerals, phytonutrients, and fiber, which serve to feed the body and cleanse the digestive tract that contains most of the body's immune system.

Amaranth greens (callaloo), avocado, bell peppers, chayote (Mexican squash), cucumber, dandelion greens, garbanzo beans (chickpeas), green banana, izote (cactus leaf), kale, lettuce (except iceberg), mushrooms (except shitake), nopales, okra, olives, onions, purslane (verdolaga), poke salad, sea vegetables (wakame, dulse, arame, hijiki, nori), squash, tomato (cherry and plum only), tomatillo, turnip greens, watercress, zucchini

OILS

It is best to minimize the use of oils because they are not a whole food, and using too much oil can lead to inflammation, support the development of diabetes, and damage arteries.

Grape-seed oil (minimize use because it is high in omega-6), sesame oil, hempseed oil, avocado oil, olive oil (better not to cook with—destroys integrity of the oil at high heat), coconut oil (better not to cook with—destroys integrity of the oil at high heat.)

SEASONINGS

Achiote, basil, bay leaf, cayenne (African bird pepper), cilantro, coriander, dill, habanero, onion powder, oregano, powdered granulated seaweed (kelp, dulce, nori), pure sea salt, sage, savory, sweet basil, tarragon, thyme

HERBAL TEAS

It is better to drink herbal teas than regular teas, like green tea, because they don't contain caffeine and contain a wide range of phytonutrients that support the immune system.

Alvaca, anise, chamomile, cloves, fennel, ginger, lemongrass, red raspberry, sea-moss tea

SUGARS

As with oils, you should minimize your consumption of additive sugar. Date sugar is the best sugar to consume from a health point of view. Date sugar is simply dried and ground dates. All of its nutrients are intact (except for its water), which controls digestion of its sugar.

Pure agave syrup (from cactus) is good, but its processing can compromise its carbohydrate structure. (Grade B maple syrup and maple sugar were recommended but have been removed from the recommended food list. Some manufacturers of maple syrup and sugar often use formaldehyde to keep the hole open in the maple tree to extract the sap. Formaldehyde is toxic and can contaminate the sap.)

CHAPTER 3:

PREPARING HERBS

Think of medicinal herbs as plants with muscles. Medicinal herbs are concentrated with nutrients and phytonutrients, which I will refer to as chemical components, and are used to combat diseases and for periodic cleansing. Herbs work best with the consumption of alkaline plant foods. If you take medicinal herbs while consuming meat, dairy, processed foods, and even acidic plant foods, you will undermine the efficacy of the herbs' chemical components. The consumption of these foods introduces toxins, pathogens, hormones, and chemicals that undermine homeostasis and the healthy operation of the organs and metabolic functions in the body.

The first step in using herbs to reverse disease is to know which are the better herbs to use and which diseases they address. The next thing to consider is whether you want to take commercial encapsulated or tonic herbs, or whether you want to prepare your own herbs using whole herbs that you either grow yourself or buy in bulk. Buying encapsulated or tonic herbs is the easier way to go, because you don't have to put any work into preparing the herbs, and the dosages are supplied on the packaging. All you need to know is which herbs to buy. Though this is the easier way to go, you take more chances with the herbs actually being what they are supposed to be and with their quality. It is commonly known that herbal supplements have been tested only to find out the many times what is advertised is not what is in the package. It is more difficult to tell which herbs you are actually buying, because herbs that have been encapsulated have been ground down to a powder and are difficult to distinguish from each other.

If you are able to grow your own herbs, it is better to get your seeds from wildcrafted plants or transplant wildcrafted plants to your growing area and grow them under as natural conditions as possible without the use of synthetic fertilizers. Wildcrafted plants are plants that grow naturally in nature without human intervention. The plants grow under natural stressors that bring out the true vitality of the plants and encourage them to develop their nutrients and phytonutrients to their optimum potency. To support these plants' optimum growth within a controlled growing environment is to use the natural fertilizer nature provides.

      I have found that a good way to get nutrients into the soil to support healthy growth of plants is to gather your garbage that contains your discarded plant parts like skins, as well as discarded meals that only contain plant remains. Blend them finely with water and use this as a fertilizer. This way you recycle the plant foods and return the unused minerals back to the soil. This is what happens in nature, without the blender. Leaves and fruits fall to the ground and get naturally recycled by being absorbed back into the ground, creating a natural cycle of restoration. If you are not able to grow your own herbs, a good alternative would be to buy whole herbs in bulk.

HARVESTING MEDICINAL HERBS

Roots, leaves, buds, and flowers are generally harvested at different times to pick each part when it has its most energy and vitality.

Roots

Generally, it is better to harvest medicinal roots in the early spring or fall when more of the plant's energy is stored in the roots. During the spring and summer, the energy and nutrients stored in the roots move to the leaves and flowers. In the fall, energy and nutrients get stored in the roots again to provide nutrients to leaves and flowers during the next spring.

Leaves

Leaves are generally picked before the plant produces flowers or seeds, before the plant has to expend energy and nutrients to support the flowers and fruits while diverting energy and nutrients away from leaves. Pick mature leaves that are strong, have a vibrant color, and have little or no insect damage.

Flowers

Harvest flowers just as they begin to open. At this point the flower has been building up energy and nutrients, but they start to decline after the flower opens all the way.

Drying Herbs

If you don't intend to use the medicinal herbs right away after you harvest them, you should dry them to protect them and to keep their nutrients intact. Traditional methods of drying herbs include making small bundles of the herbs and hanging them from a clothesline, with a couple of inches between each bundle to allow air to circulate and dry out the herbs. The area where you dry the herbs should not be humid, because that will help keep water in the plants instead of pulling the water out. The area should not be in direct sunlight so that it doesn't initiate chemical reactions in herbs that can compromise their quality. Instead of hanging the herbs from a clothesline, you can also lay out the herbs on a screen, spaced apart so the herbs can get good airflow. The screens should be hung or should sit on supports to raise them from surfaces to allow air to move up and down through the screens freely.

You can also use a dehydrator to dry the herbs, which will quicken the drying process. The important thing to remember is you want to keep the temperature between 90° and 105°F to maintain the quality of the nutrients and phytonutrients.

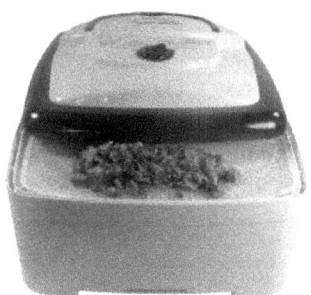

After the herbs have dried, store the whole herbs in glass jars with airtight or tight-fitting lids. Allowing air to circulate on the herbs will reduce the potency of the herbs' components over time. Store the herbs in a cool, dark, and dry place to retain the herbs' medicinal potency for a longer period.

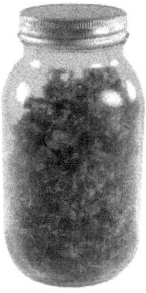

BULK HERBS

Instead of harvesting your own herbs, you can also opt to purchase whole herbs in bulk. This would be a better option than purchasing prepackaged encapsulated herbs, though the capsules are the easiest to use. Buying bulk herbs gives you a better idea of what you are actually purchasing, because you get to examine the herb to determine if it is what it is supposed to be. You can compare it to what you have seen or to pictures.

Bulk herb packages usually consist of whole herbs, but sometimes they consist of ground or powdered herbs. For quality control, it is better to buy whole herbs or pieces of herbs and grind them into a powder. When you are ready to use some of the herb, grind down a small portion. You can encapsulate the herbs in vegetable capsules and store the capsules in a container. You can store the ground herb directly in a glass jar with an airtight or tight-fitting lid. To protect the medicinal compounds in the herbs, it is better to store them in a cool, dark, and dry place.

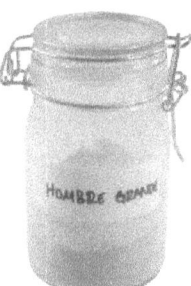

Storing a ground herb in and airtight container preserves its medicinal value

Bulk herbs are purchased from herbal distributors more often come in sixteen-ounce packages. You can also find herbs in eight-ounce and four-ounce packages, and sometimes even two-ounce packages. You will find most bulk herbs sold as whole herbs are pieces of herbs, while a few bulk herbs are sold powdered.

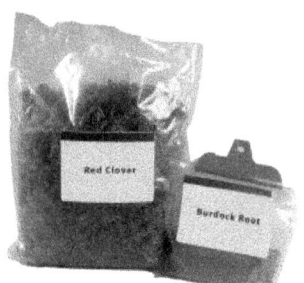

MAKING HERBS

You can make medicinal herbs by breaking down whole herbs into smaller parts or by using various extraction methods to remove chemical compounds from the herbs. This extraction method discards the fiber and components bound to the fiber, so in most cases I prefer to use whole herb, grind it down to encapsulate it, or drink the ground herb with water. The extraction method is used to get the chemical components into the bloodstream quickly, because the body will not have to spend time breaking down the herbs to remove the chemical compounds from the fiber. This has its positive side and its drawback. Using medicinal herbs this way is good in flooding the bloodstream with chemical components, but this is also a little too good.

The kidneys work hard to maintain the delicate balance of minerals, water, and other compounds, and a rush of chemical components into the bloodstream forces the kidneys to pass some of them to the bladder and out of the body. In contrast, grinding down the herbs into finer particles allows the body to access more of the herbs' chemicals in a more controlled manner.

You don't want to consume large pieces of herbs, because intact plant cell walls resist being broken down. The herbs' chemical compounds are stored within the cell walls of the leaf, flower, root, bark, or seed. Consuming large or whole pieces of herbs will result in less nutrients being released and absorbed into the bloodstream, which is why it is important to thoroughly chew your food.

It would be pretty difficult to properly chew raw leaves, flowers, roots, bark, and seeds and thoroughly break down their cells walls and release most of their nutrients.

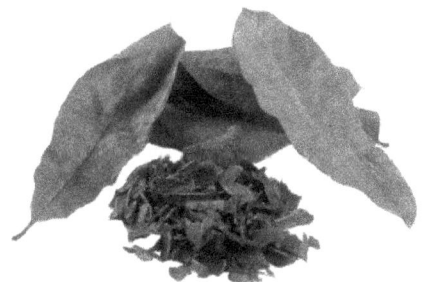

Grinding down herbs into powder or fine particles allows the body to access more of their nutrients.

Grinding down herbs into smaller particles allows the digestive process access to much more of the herbs' compounds, and at a quicker rate. Maintaining all of their fiber and compounds controls digestion, so the bloodstream is not spiked with nutrients, resulting in an unbalance of minerals and components in the bloodstream. Grinding down herbs offers faster digestion and absorption of nutrients into the bloodstream than consuming large portions of whole herbs does. This speeds up but still controls the herbs' digestion, in contrast to consuming the extracted compounds from herbs, so more of the nutrients are actually used by the body.

Sometimes medicinal herb extractions are preferable in the form of infusions or decoctions when it comes to certain herbs, or when performing general maintenance.

INFUSION

Infusions are medicinal herbs whose chemicals have been removed by steeping leaves, buds, flowers, berries, and some seeds of plants in boiling water. Infusions are made with the softer parts of plants, because steeping them in hot water is enough to adequately penetrate the herb's cell walls. Infusing the softer parts of the plants will allow the release of a good portion of the herb's components into the water.

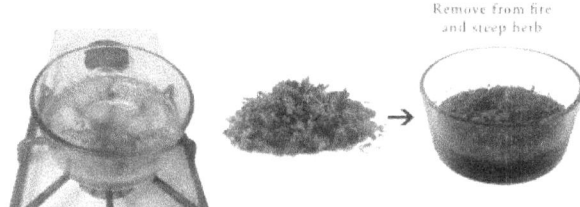

Preparation

1. 1 tablespoon of dried herb or 1½ tablespoons of fresh herb.
2. Boil 8 ounces and remove from fire.
3. Add herb to the water. Let steep for 30 to 45 minutes. (The longer you let the herb steep, the more chemical components will be extracted while the water is hot. The darker or more colored the water becomes, the more components are released from the herb, and the stronger the infusion will be.)
4. Strain the infusion and drink.

Multiply the tablespoon of herb and the ounces of water by the same number to increase the amount of infusion. If you use 4 tablespoons of herb you would use 32 ounces of water.

DECOCTION

Decoctions are similar to infusions, but they use the tougher parts of the plant like the roots, twigs, and bark. Since these parts of the plant are harder and tougher, pouring boiling water on them will release only a small amount of the herb's components. Decoctions involve boiling and simmering these parts of the plant to more effectively remove their chemicals.

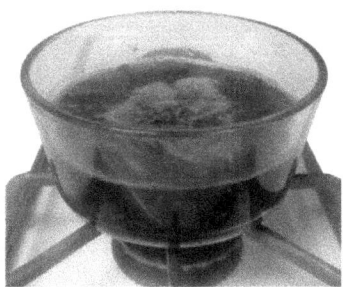

Preparation

1. 1 tablespoon of dried herb or 1½ tablespoons of fresh herb.
2. 8 ounces of water and herb to saucepan.
3. Bring the water to a boil in a covered pot, reduce heat, and simmer on low setting for 30 minutes. More components are extracts the longer the water is simmered.
4. Let the water cool and add the mixture to a mason jar.

Follow the instructions for the infusion to increase the amount of the decoction.

GRINDING HERBS, ENCAPSULATION, AND DOSAGE

Grinding

The better way to gain all the benefits of an herb is to consume the ground whole herb. For the more delicate parts of the plants, like the leaves, buds, flowers, and some seeds, a simple coffee grinder will be able to sufficiently grind these parts into finer particles that the body can more easily digest.

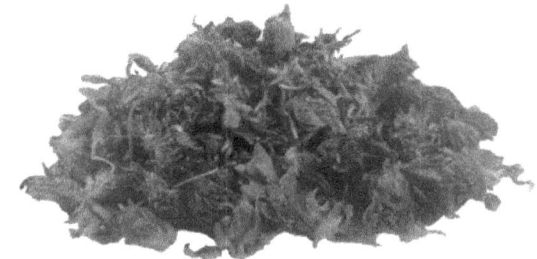

Dried buds, flowers and leaves

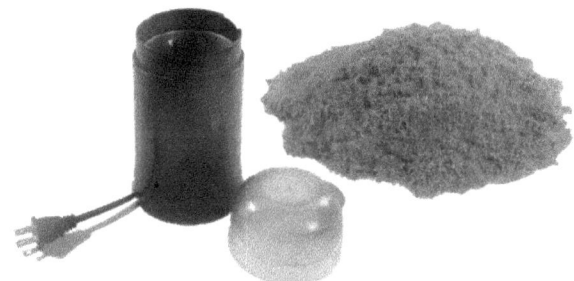

Inexpensive bladed coffee grinders are able to grind leaves, buds, flowers and seeds with relative ease. Ground buds, flowers, and leaves.

For harder parts like twigs, branches, roots, and bark, you will need an industrial grinder or a heavy-duty industrial blender. Industrial grinders will be able to grind down the very hard parts of the plants into powder with more ease. Industrial blenders are also able to grind down the harder part of the plants but take a little bit longer, though they can grind down the herbs to less fine particles more easily.

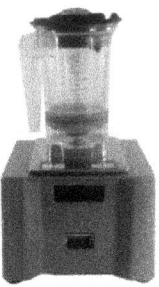

Industrial blender and accessory jar used for grinding beans and grains into flower. The smaller jar is more suitable for grinding herbs.

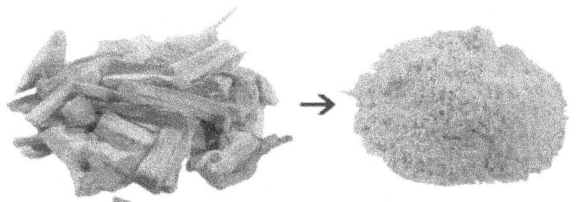

Wood chips turned into a powder with an industrial blender.

Encapsulation

You can buy cheap encapsulation kits which make encapsulating herbs pretty easy. Cap M Quik makes kits for "0", "00", and "000" size capsules. I use "00" kit with vegetarian capsules. Filled "00" capsules contain around 500 mg of herb.

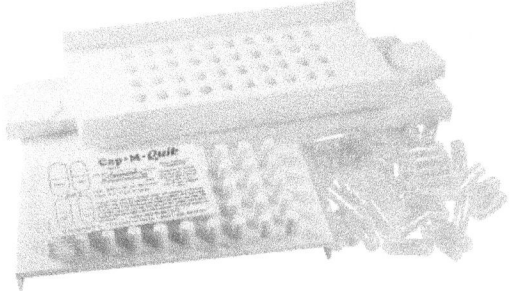

Cap M Quik kit and "00" vegetarian capsules

Dosage

The general dosages for herbs are based on an adult person around 150 pounds. The maximum recommended dosage for an herbal extract for an adult person around 150 pounds is six grams per day. This dosage is often applied to the whole herbs also, though herbal extracts are more concentrated in chemical compounds. The dosage of herb per capsule is around five hundred milligrams or half a gram. So the maximum dosage for capsules that contain around five hundred milligrams of a particular herb is twelve capsules daily.

The concern for exact dosage is generally more stringent for pharmaceutical medicine than for herbal medicine, and for good reason. Around 50 percent of pharmaceutical medicines are derived from plants, but the difference is that pharmaceutical medicine isolates the active compound from a plant and concentrates it or duplicates it synthetically. The concentration of the active ingredient is far more potent and dangerous than herbal medicine, because the amount of the active ingredient going into the body is abnormally high, and since the active ingredient is isolated, it doesn't have the other nutrients of the plant to control its digestion. Though the pharmaceutical medicine is based on something natural, it isn't natural and has a different effect in the body. Herbal medicine is far more forgiving, but that doesn't mean you should intentionally take abnormally high dosages of herbs. Too much of anything overwhelms that natural processes of the body.

When you look at the dosages for herbs on commercial bottled herbal products, the dosages are generally around two or three capsules, two or three times a day. Capsules generally contain around five hundred milligrams of herb, so the maximum dosage of nine capsules a day would be 4500 mg or 4.5 g a day. This is still far below the recommended dosage. If you are using loose herbs instead of capsules, one capsule is approximately a quarter teaspoon. Two or three capsules would be equivalent to one-half to three-quarters of a teaspoon, and at two or three times daily, the maximum dosage would be two and one-quarter teaspoons of herb daily.

This dosage is for a single herb, but in herbal medicine, herbs are often combined to address a particular condition, clean a specific organ, or support a specific function. Different herbs contain different chemical compounds that address the same condition or situation in different ways. Though the chemical compounds are different, the dosages are often reduced for each herb to stay within the maximum recommended daily dosage of six grams per day, or the maximum of nine daily commercial herbal capsules.

This information is intended to give a better understanding of how herbs and dosages are prepared, for educational purposes. Though some people will use this information to help better their understanding in preparing herbs themselves, it is also important to understand that herbalists spend a lot of time learning about herbs and how to prepare medicinal herbs, and they have a better understanding of the particular nuances that are involved in preparing them. Herbalists will have a better understanding of combining herbs and adjusting their dosage.

If you were combining herbs and each one used the same dosage, then determining the dose for the combined herbs would be pretty straightforward. You would take one part of each herb and thoroughly mix them together. You would either encapsulate the mixed herbs and follow the dosages generally recommended by commercial herbal products, or measure out the equivalent amount of loose herb and drink it with water or a vegetable or fruit smoothie. Some nuances you will need to know how to address include knowing how many or the maximum amount of herbs to combine so that you do not use too little of a particular herb and reduce its effectiveness.

A general recommendation is to use four or five herbs at a maximum when combining herbs to address a particular issue, and if you use more herbs, then you may need to increase the dosage. An herbalist would have more experience in this situation to make an educated decision in increasing the dosage. Another complication is that some herbs are used at a lower dosage than the general recommended dosage, and this adds another wrinkle to combining herbs and determining the dose for each herb.

CHILDREN'S DOSAGES

Determining children's dosages of herbs may be a daunting task, but it shouldn't be. Many people are scared to administer natural herbs, which are just different parts of plants, to their children, but are comfortable administering pharmaceutical medicines, which are dangerous and cause numerous deaths every year. There is something really problematic with this paradigm. Determining dosages of herbs for children is pretty simple, and there are formulas that are used to determine the dosage.

Clarke's Rule

Clarke's rule can be found in *Pharmaceutical Calculations*,[19] by Howard C. Ansel. To determine the child's dosage, you will need to know the child's weight and the adult dosage. If the capsule contains five hundred milligrams of herb and the dosage calls for two capsules, the adult dose would be one thousand milligrams or one gram. If the child's weight is seventy pounds, you calculate the dose using the Clarke's rule.

$$\frac{\text{Weight of child (in lbs)} \times \text{Adult dose}}{150 \text{ (average weight of adult in lbs)}} = \text{Child's Dose}$$

$$\frac{70 \times 1000 \text{ mg}}{150} = 467 \text{ mg}$$

In this case the child's dose would be around half of the adult dose.

If you are being helped by an herbalist, it is still good to understand of how herbs are selected and how dosages are applied, because the knowledge will allow you to ask educated questions. The same approach should be taken when dealing with a medical doctor. Though you may need help from a more qualified person, your health is ultimately your responsibility, and you should have some understanding of what you are being given. The mind is also a very important player in the process of healing. Understanding what a particular herb does and knowing that it is being applied correctly leads to a confidence that the herb will work, and this multiplies the herb's efficacy.

CHAPTER 4:

ALKALINE MEDICINAL HERBS

The alkaline movement is running strong, thanks to the work of the herbalist Dr. Sebi, who has spearheaded the alkaline movement with his African Bio Mineral Balance. Many herbalists use many various herbs to reverse disease. Dr. Sebi has been instrumental in identifying the natural alkaline herbs from these that best support the healthy expression of the African genome that is the foundation of all people.

These herbs are herbs whose chemical composition hasn't been compromised through hybridization and genetic modification. The herbs that have mostly developed in environments of Africa or similar to Africa, under the same conditions as the African genome, have chemical affinity with it. These herbs help promote an environment of ease within the body that supports physical, mental, emotional, and spiritual stability and rejuvenation in all people.

These herbs serve as a foundation for healing and reversing disease. Though Dr. Sebi's list of herbs that best support the African genome is not exhaustive, these herbs are differentiated from many other commonly used herbs that are hybrid and acidic in nature. Though these other herbs do have some beneficial properties, they also introduce compounds that don't have chemical affinity with the body, cause issues with homeostasis, and reduce the herb's efficacy. Herbs like comfrey and even the popular echinacea fall into this category because of their incomplete chemical structure due to hybridization, genetic, or biological manipulation.

I will address the alkaline herbs Dr. Sebi uses to reverse disease, which have been used for hundreds, if not thousands, of years in traditional medicine. I would also be remiss to not identify a few herbs that may not be part of Dr. Sebi's list but that are indigenous to areas that are similar to the environment of

Africa, like the guinea hen weed of Jamaica.

HERBS AND THEIR PROPERTIES

(For educational purposes only. This information has not been evaluated by the Food and Drug Administration. This information is not intended to diagnose, treat, cure, or prevent any disease.) The general dosages listed are for using single herbs, and the general dosages for herbal combinations are explained in the next chapter.

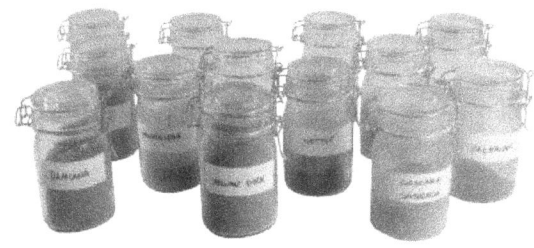

Arnica

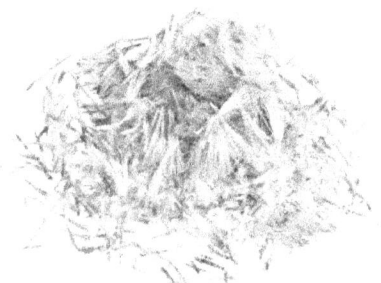

Arnica (*Arnica montana*, Radix Ptarmicae Montanae, arnica flowers, mountain tobacco) is a powerful anti-inflammatory and antiseptic herb. It is used primarily to treat external wounds, and it relieves pain and promotes tissue regeneration. Arnica is used externally in the form of creams and compresses to treat arthritis, sprains, bruises, and headaches. Arnica infusions are used for its antiseptic properties to clean wounds, abscesses, and boils. Dr. Sebi uses arnica as part of his **uterine wash** compound.

Origin: North America General commercial dose: Arnica is used primarily as a topical cream.

(Medical caution: For external use only. Arnica may be toxic when ingested orally, often leading to severe irritation of mucous membranes and the gastrointestinal tract.)

Batana

Batana oil (*Elaeis oleifera*, American oil palm, palm oil) is made from the kernel of the fruit of the *Elaeis oleifera* tree. The oil is used primarily for its fatty acids, nutrients, and phytonutrients as a hair oil to strengthen hair, to promote its growth, and as a natural hair coloring. It naturally turns gray hair brown.

Origin: Honduras, Central and South America

Bladderwrack

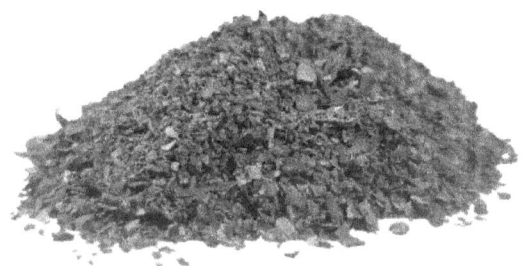

Bladderwrack (*Fucus vesiculosus*, fucus) is used primarily because it is a high source of iodine. Bladderwrack has been used traditionally to treat an underactive and oversized thyroid and to treat iodine deficiency. Bladderwrack is also rich in calcium, magnesium, and potassium, and it contains other trace minerals. Bladderwrack contains numerous phytonutrients, which are credited with its many health benefits. Fucoxanthin anchors its antioxidant benefits.[20] Bladderwrack has antiestrogenic effects and has been shown to lower the risk of estrogen-dependent diseases.[21],[22] Bladderwrack lowers lipid and cholesterol levels[23] and supports weight loss. Its mucopolysaccharide phytonutrients inhibit skin enzymes from breaking down in the skin, reduce skin thickness, and improve elasticity.[24] Bladderwrack has also shown anticandida, antibacterial,[25],[26] and antitumor properties.[27]

Bladderwrack is used as a natural **iodine supplement**, and one 580 mg capsule contains around 155 percent of iodine's recommended daily value. It is interesting that the Japanese intake of iodine is 1000–3000 mcg per day without any side effects.[28]

Origin: Atlantic Ocean, Pacific Ocean, North Sea, Baltic Sea General commercial dose: One 580 mg capsule General dosage: One capsule daily

Blessed Thistle

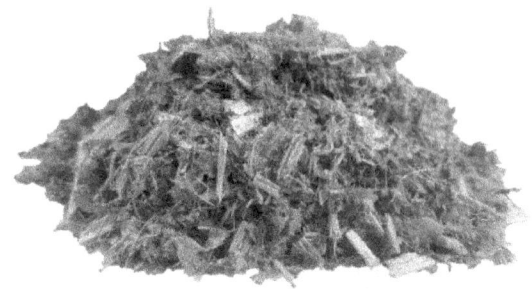

Blessed thistle (*Cnicus benedictus*, cardo santo, centaurea benedicta, folia cardui benedicti, holy thistle) belongs to the Asteraceae plant family. Blessed thistle is high in iron and has been used in traditional medicine to increase circulation and oxygen delivery to the brain, to support brain function, and to support heart and lung function. Its bitter phytonutrients are used to support liver and gallbladder function and to stimulate the upper digestive tract to promote proper digestion and improve appetite.[29],[30],[31]

Blessed thistle has antifungal and diuretic properties and has been used traditionally for its emmenagogue properties that treat hormonal disorders that interfere with normal menstruation. Blessed thistle is also considered a galactagogue and has been used to increase and enrich milk flow in nursing mothers. Blessed thistle is also used to remove toxins, acids, and mucus and to assist in **intracellular cleansing** (inside cells).

Origin: Mediterranean General commercial dose: One 390mg capsule General dosage: Two capsules three times daily *(Medical caution: women who are pregnant or nursing are advised to consult a health-care professional before use. Persons with allergies to plants of the Asteraceae family should use with caution.)*

Blue Vervain

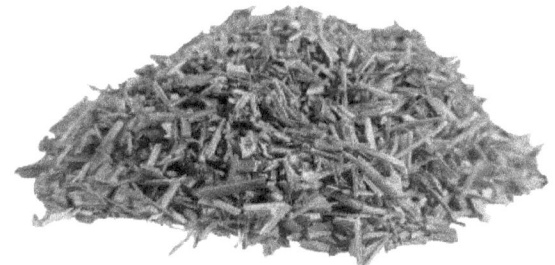

Blue vervain (*Verbena hastate*, simpler's joy, verbena) has diuretic, antimalarial,[32] anti-inflammatory,[33] and antimicrobial[34] properties. Blue vervain has been used in traditional medicine as a female tonic to treat menstrual cramps[35] and as an emmenagogue[36] to increase milk production in women who are breastfeeding. A primary use of blue vervain is to treat **nervous disorders** including, stress, anxiety, and restlessness.[37]

Origin: North America General commercial dose: One 400 mg capsule General dosage: One capsule two times daily

Burdock Root

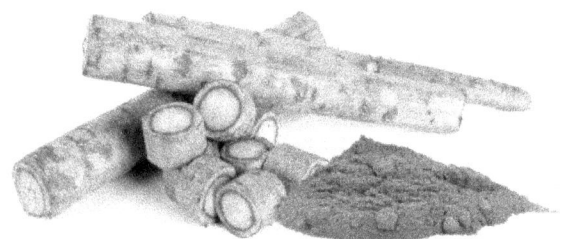

Burdock root (*Arctium lappa*) is also known as bardana. Burdock root is a diuretic, blood cleanser, anti-inflammatory, antioxidant,[38] antifungus, anticancer,[39] antiviral, and antibacterial herb.[40] Many of burdock root's medicinal properties are attributed to its wide array of chemical compounds, which include inulin, mucilage, essential oil, volatile oil, alkaloids, glycosides, resin, and tannins. Burdock has been used in traditional medicine to treat skin conditions such as eczema, acne, and psoriasis, because it promotes the removal of toxins from the skin. It is also a diuretic used promote urination to stimulate kidney function and repair. A primary use of burdock root is as a blood purifier and liver tonic to restore **liver function** and health.

Origin: Africa, Asia, Europe General commercial dose: One 500 mg capsule General dosage: Two capsules three times daily

Cascara Sagrada

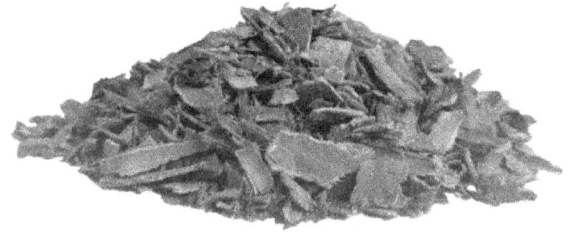

Cascara sagrada (*Rhamnus purshiana*, sacred bark, pushiana, purschiana bark, persiana bark, chittam bark) contains emodin, which has antiviral and anticancer properties.[41],[42] Cascara sagrada is used primarily as a laxative and **stimulates the peristaltic action of the intestine**. This wavelike motion moves waste through the intestine. This property helps restore the proper tone and health of the intestine by **pushing waste out of diverticula pouches** that develop in the intestinal wall. This helps **restore the mucous lining and health of the intestine**. Cascara sagrada has been used in traditional medicine to improve stomach, liver, and pancreas secretions and to break up and remove gallstones from the gallbladder.

Origin: Western North America General commercial dose: One 450 mg capsule General dosage: One or two capsules, preferably at bedtime *(Medical caution: do not use if you have or develop diarrhea or abdominal pain. Women who are pregnant or nursing are advised avoid cascara sagrada because it can induce labor, and lactating women can pass on the compound via breastfeeding. Not recommended for longer than seven consecutive days. It is very important to not exceed recommended doses to avoid liver damage. Cascara sagrada use has been shown to be safe and useful within recommended usage.)*

Chaparral

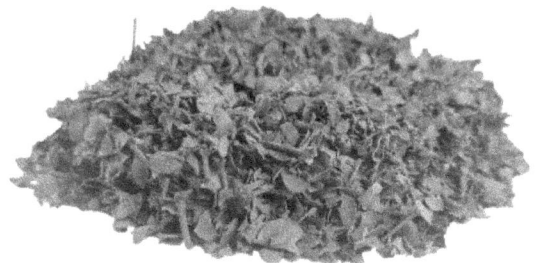

Chaparral (*Larrea tridentate*, goverrnadora) has antimicrobial and antibacterial,[43] antitumor and anticancer,[44] and antiulcerogenic and anti-inflammatory properties.[45] Traditionally, chaparral has been used to kill parasites; address sexually transmitted diseases; treat skin conditions like eczema, psoriasis, skin rashes, and bruises; and as an expectorant to treat respiratory issues like colds and bronchitis.

Origin: Mexico, Southwest North America General commercial dose: One 500 mg capsule General dosage: One capsule two times daily *(Medical caution: on rare occasions high doses have been shown to contribute liver disease, but recommended doses have been shown to be safe.)*

Cocolmeca

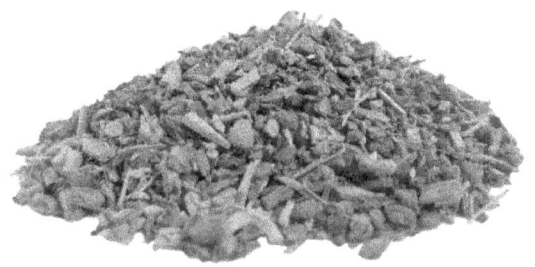

Cocolmeca (*Smilax, Smilax regelii, Smilax aristolochiifolia*, Jamaican sarsaparilla cocolmeca bark, cuculmeca) has anti-inflammatory, antiulcer, antioxidant,[46] anticancer,[47] diaphoretic, and diuretic properties. Cocolmeca is a plant of the *Smilax* genus and has been shown to bind with toxins for their removal from the blood and body.[48] Cocolmeca is used in traditional medicine to treat skin conditions like psoriasis and leprosy, rheumatoid arthritis and joint pain, headaches, colds, and sexual impotence.

Origin: Mexico, Jamaica General commercial dose: One 450 mg capsule General dosage: One capsule two times daily

Contribo

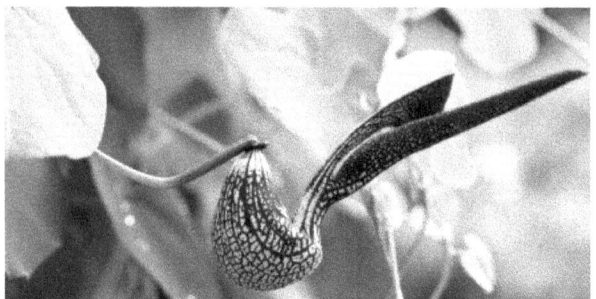

Contribo (*Aristolochia, Aristolochia grandiflora*, birthwort, duckflower, alcatraz, hierba del Indio) is used in traditional medicine for arthritis and edema, to stimulate the immune system and white-blood-cell production, to kill parasites, and to treat snakebites.

Origin: South America General commercial dose: Not used in commercial products (found to be poisonous) *(Medical caution: women who are pregnant or nursing should avoid contribo. Contribo is cited as being toxic to the kidneys and should be used only under strict, knowledgeable supervision.)*

Damiana

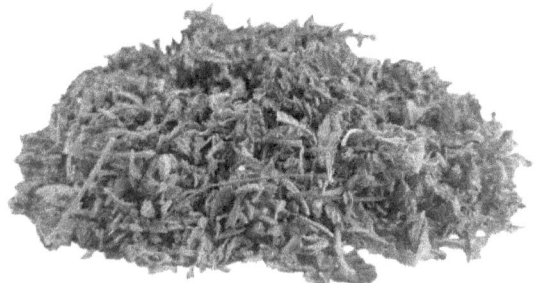

Damiana (*Turnera diffusa*, turnera, turnea aprodisiaca, damiana aphrodisiaca, damiana herb, damiana leaf) has anti-aromatase[49] and antianxiety[50] properties. B men and women use damiana to **strengthen the sexual organs** and boost sexual drive and potency. The anti-aromatase property blocks androstenedione and estrone conversion to estrogen. Damiana is used to help control estrogen related illness in women like breast cancer and fibroids. Women also use it to reduce hot flashes associated with menopause. It also helps balance estrogen and supports testosterone levels in men. Damiana increases oxygen delivery to the genitals, resulting in increased libido.[51],[52] Damiana is also used to treat depression and nervousness and to relieve anxiety associated with sexual dysfunction. Damiana stimulates the intestinal tract and is used to treat constipation.

Origin: Mexico, Central and South America, the Caribbean General commercial dose: One 400 mg capsule General dosage: Two capsules two or three times daily

Elderberry

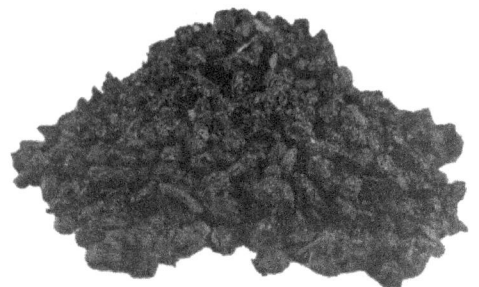

Elderberry (*Sambucus, Sambucus nigra, Sambucus africana*) has anti-inflammatory, antiviral, anti-influenza, and anticancer properties. It is used to treat colds, the flu, and allergies and to **remove mucus** from the respiratory system. *Sambucus nigra* is most commonly used medicinally because it has been shown to be nontoxic, while other species can be toxic. *Sambucus nigra* has been shown in studies to bind with the H1N1 virus[53] and stop it from entering cells.

Origin: America, Africa, Asia, Europe General commercial dose: One 500 mg capsule General dosage: Two capsules two or three times daily

Eyebright

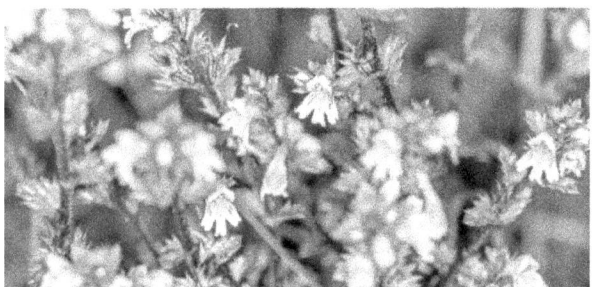

Eyebright (*Euphrasia officinalis*, *Euphrasia rostkoviana*) has anti-inflammatory and antiseptic properties and is used to as an **eyewash** to sooth the eye's mucous membrane and to treat chronic inflammation of the eye. Eyebright is used as an antimicrobial to treat the conjunctivitis and blepharitis bacterial infections of the eye.[54] Eyebright is used as an astringent to treat wounds and reduce skin inflammation. It is also used internally as an anti-inflammatory to treat upper respiratory infections like sinusitis and hay fever.

Origin: ~

General commercial dose: One 450 mg capsule General dosage: Two capsules once daily Eyewash: Steep ½ teaspoon of eyebright herb in 8 oz. of boiled water for 15 minutes. Strain through cheesecloth into a container to remove herb particles. Use an eyewash cup to wash the eyes.

Place the eyewash cup over the eye you want to clean. Tilt your head back a little so the wash covers the entire eye. For 20 seconds rotate your eye right to left and up and down. After you are done cleaning one eye, discard the eyewash, refill the eyewash cup, and then clean the second eye.

Wash two times daily.

Guaco

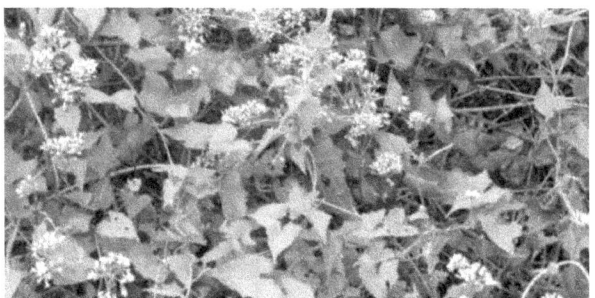

Guaco (*Mikania guaco, Mikania glomerata,* guace, bejuco de finca, cepu, liane francois, matafinca, vedolin, cipó caatinga, huaco, erva das serpentes) has anti-inflammatory,[55] antiallergic,[56] and bronchodilator[57],[58] properties. Guaco is used primarily in traditional medicine for **upper respiratory problems** like asthma, bronchitis, colds, and flu. It is used as an anti-inflammatory agent for rheumatoid arthritis and inflammation in the digestive tract[59] and as an antibacterial for Candida and yeast infections. Guaco contains around 10 percent coumarin, which has blood-thinning properties.

Origin: South America, Jamaica General dose: Guaco is usually consumed as an infusion/tea— 4 oz. standard infusion. Standard infusion: 1 tablespoon herb to 1 cup/8 oz. of boiling water. Steep the herb in the boiling water for 15–20 minutes.

General dosage: 4 oz. two or three times daily General commercial dose: One 300 mg capsule General dosage: One capsule two or three times daily

(Medical caution: consult with your physician before taking this plant if you are taking coumarin/coumadin drugs or if coumarin/coumadin anticoagulant-type drugs are contraindicated for your condition.)

Huereque

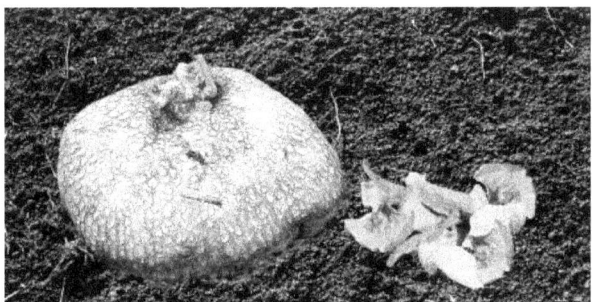

Huereque (*Ibervillea sonorae*, guareque, wareki, choyalhuani, wereke, big root, coyote melon, cowpie plant) has hypoglycemic,[60] antiobesity,[61] and antimicrobial[62] properties. Huereque is used in traditional medicine to lower blood-sugar levels, **treat diabetes**, and reduce weight. It is used to nourish and **cleanse the pancreas**.

Origin: Northwest Mexico General commercial dose: One 500 mg capsule General dosage: One capsule three times daily with meals

Hombre Grande

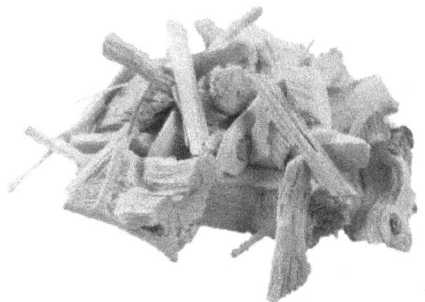

Hombre grande (*Picrasma excelsa, Quassia amara* L., quassia, cuassia mara, Jamaican quassia, amargo, bitter ash, bitter bark, bitter wood) has antifungal, antiulcer,[63] antimalarial,[64] anticancer,[65] and insecticide properties. Hombre grande has been used in traditional medicine topically to treat measles and orally to treat constipation and diarrhea, intestinal parasite infections, and fever. It is used to stimulate the digestive tract and bile production, increase appetite, cleanse blood, and stimulate enzyme production. Hombre grande helps rebalance the flora in the digestive tract to support the **immune system**.

Origin: The Caribbean, Jamaica, Central and South America General commercial dose: One 450 mg capsule General dosage: One capsule three times daily (Traditionally this herb was made into a tincture because it is made from the bark of the plant. Grinders are used now to make a powder that can be taken in capsule form or in hot water.) *(Medical caution: not recommended for women who are pregnant. Antifertility properties have been shown to reduce testes size and sperm size in a laboratory setting. Men who are* planning to make a baby should avoid using hombre grande. [66] *You should not take* hombre grande beyond the recommended dosage or for a long, continuous amount of time.*)*

Hops

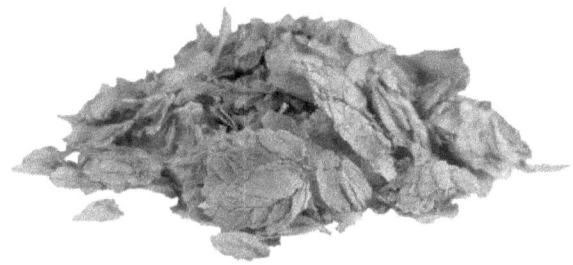

Hops (*Humulus lupulus*, lupulo) has antibacterial, anti-inflammatory, and anticancer properties.[67] Hops is used in traditional medicine to **break up inflammation**; relieve pain; promote digestion, urination, and appetite; treat rheumatic pains, infections, insomnia and sleeping disorders; and reduce anxiety, tension, attention deficit hyperactivity disorder (ADHD), irritability, and **nervousness**.

Origin: Germany General commercial dose: One 310 mg capsule General dosage: Two capsules once daily or one capsule twice daily

Hydrangea

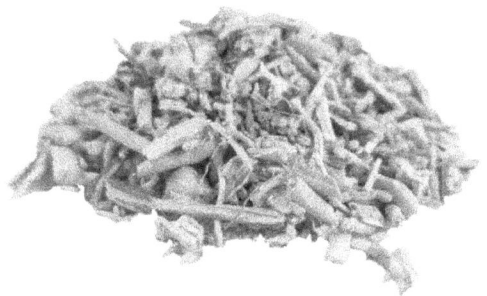

Hydrangea Root (*Hydrangea*, *Hydrangea arborescens*, hortensia, seven barks) has anti-inflammatory,[68] lithotrophic, antiseptic, antiparasitic, and autoimmune properties. Hydrangea is used for its hydrangin compound, which **dissolves calcium deposits in soft tissue**. It has been used traditionally to treat bladder and kidney disease, to **dissolve kidney stones**, and to clean the lymphatic system. Chang Shan is used in Chinese medicine for its febriugine compound to treat autoimmune diseases.[69]

Origin: Northeastern Asia, Southwestern United States General commercial dose: One 400 mg capsule General dosage: Two capsules two times daily

Lavender

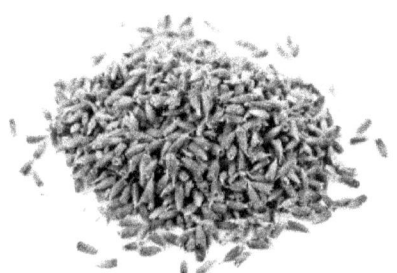

Lavender (*Lavandula*) has antifungal,[70] antibacterial,[71],[72] analgesic, anti-inflammatory,[73] anti-insomnia, anticonvulsant, antispasmodic,[74] and antianxiety and antidepressant[75],[76] properties. Lavender is used is traditional medicine to treat restlessness, insomnia, **nervousness**, and depression. Lavender is used for migraines, nerve pain, and joint pain. It is also used to reverse abdominal swelling from gas, upset stomach, nausea, loss of appetite, and vomiting.

Origin: Africa, Canary Islands, Mediterranean, Asia, India Lavender is used mostly as an essential oil and is made through distillation. This will leave you with pure lavender oil, but it takes around 150 parts of lavender to make 1 part oil. (It would take around 150 oz. of lavender to make 1 oz. of oil.) The distilled lavender is primarily used for inhalation.

You can make a cold infusion of lavender by adding crushed fresh dried lavender to a jar and adding enough oil to cover it. (Coconut oil would add to its medicinal properties.) Don't fill the jar completely so you leave room for air in the jar. Put the jar in a sunny location. You should smell the lavender in the oil after forty-eight hours, but the oil is usually left in the sun for up to six weeks. The lavender infusion is used as cologne or perfume, or as a rubbing oil for soreness and arthritis. Lavender is also consumed as a ground.

General commercial dose: One 500 mg capsule General dosage: One capsule one to three times daily

Lily of the Valley

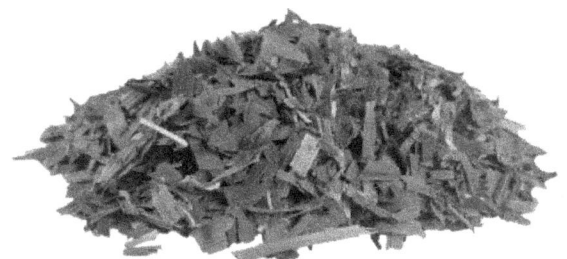

Lily of the valley (*Convallaria majalis*, clochette des bois, constancy, convallaria, convallaria herba, convall-lily, gazon de parnasse, Jacob's ladder, ladder-to-heaven, our lady's tears) has antiangiogenic, antitumor,[77] and diuretic properties. Lily of the valley has been used for hundreds of years in traditional medicine primarily as a **heart tonic** to treat heart failure and irregular heartbeat. Lily of the valley's action is similar to the drug Digitalis, but it is natural, less concentrated, and therefore less powerful. It is used to treat heart debility and dropsy. It promotes increased oxygen delivery to the heart, reduces blood pressure, and relaxes a weak heart to beat more slowly and efficiently while increasing its power.

Origin: Europe, Northern Asia

General dose: 1 tablespoon of infusion daily (It is difficult to find a commercial bottled product, because lily of the valley is administered by a professional herbalist or medical practitioner.

An infusion of lily of the valley is made from adding from ½
oz. of the herb to one pint of boiling water. The infusion is allowed to steep until it is cool. It is stored preferably in an airtight glass container in a cool, dark place.

It is better not to strain the herb, but to shake the mixture and use a tablespoon of the mixture.)

(Medical caution: should be used only under professional supervision. Lily of the valley shouldn't be taken with pharmaceutical medicines and can interfere with heart medications. Not recommended for

women who are pregnant.)

Nettle

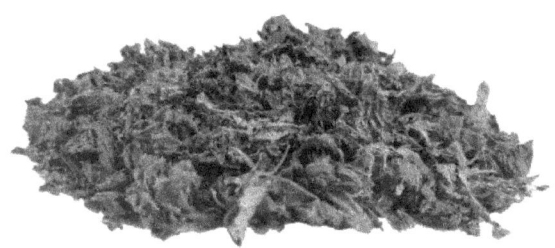

Nettle (*Urtica dioica*, ortiga, stinging nettle) has anti-inflammatory, anticancer, [78] diuretic, antioxidant, antimicrobial, antiulcer, and analgesic activities. [79] Nettle root is used for an enlarged prostate, for joints, and as a diuretic and astringent. Nettle leaves are used for arthritis, sore muscles, hair loss, anemia, poor circulation, diabetes, enlarged spleen, allergies, eczema and rash, and asthma. Nettle is used as a general **health tonic** and **blood purifier**.

Origin: North Africa, Asia, Western North America **Nettle Leaf** General commercial dose: One 435 mg capsule General dosage: Two capsules two times daily **Nettle Root** General commercial dose: One 400 mg capsule General dosage: Two capsules one or two times daily *(Medical caution: women who are pregnant should consult with a physician.)*

Nopal

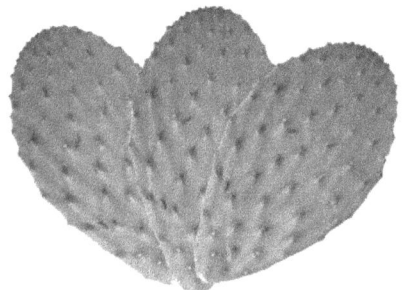

Nopal (*Opuntia*, prickly pear, nopal cactus) is the paddle of the *Opuntia* cactus, which also produces the prickly-pear fruit. Nopal contains numerous phytochemicals, antioxidants, vitamins, and minerals. It is used to reverse type 2 diabetes, high cholesterol, obesity, alcohol hangover, colitis, diarrhea, and viral infections.

Origin: Mexico, Central America, the Caribbean, Western United States, Eastern United States General commercial dose: One 400 mg capsule General dosage: Two capsules two times daily

Prodigiosa

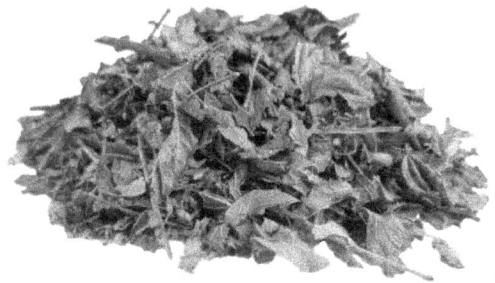

Prodigiosa (*Brickellia canvanillesi*, prodigiosa, amula, hamula, calea zacatechichi, dream herb, cheech, bitter grass) is used in traditional medicine to **stimulate pancreas** and **liver** secretions, increasing bile synthesis and evacuation of bile from the gallbladder. Prodigiosa is used to treat diarrhea, stomach pain, and gallbladder disease, and it is used to treat **diabetes**[80],[81], [82] by controlling blood-sugar levels. Prodigiosa is used to treat **headaches** and fever. Prodigiosa has antianxiety[83] properties and induces a **vivid dream** state.

Origin: Southwestern North America, New Mexico General dose: Prodigiosa is usually consumed as a infusion/tea—2–4 oz. standard infusion. Standard infusion: 1
tablespoon herb to 1 cup/8 oz. of boiling water. Steep the herb in the boiling water for 15–20 minutes.[84]

General dosage: Two times daily—morning and evening Suggested capsule dose: One 400 mg capsule Suggested capsule dosage: One capsule two times daily (Start at a lower dose if necessary) *(Medical caution: women who are pregnant should consult with a physician. People with type 1 diabetes are advised to consult with a physician. Do not exceed suggested dosage.)*

Red Clover

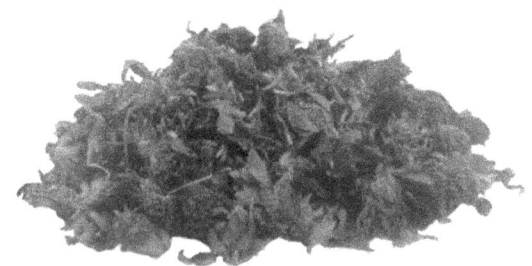

Red clover (*Trifolium pratense*, meadow honeysuckle, meadow trefoil, purple clover, trefoil, wild clover, cleaver grass, marl grass, cow grass) has anticancer, [85] diuretic, expectorant, and sedative, anti-inflammatory, and antiatherosclerosis[86] properties. Red clover is used for its estrogen properties to relieve menopausal symptoms. Red clover is a **blood purifier** and is used to **break up calcification** in soft tissues and to **clean the lymphatic system** of lymph fluid waste.

Origin: Northwest Africa, Western Asia General commercial dose: One 400 mg capsule General dosage: Two capsules once daily or one capsule twice daily *(Medical caution: not recommended for women who are pregnant.)*

Rhubarb Root

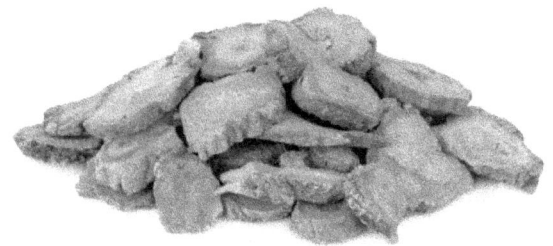

Rhubarb root (*Rheum palmatum*, Chinese rhubarb, Turkish rhubarb, Indian rhubarb, Russian rhubarb, *R. tanguticum* and *R. officinale* - da-huang) has antioxidant, heavy-metal chelation, anticancer,[87] and antibacterial[88] properties. Rhubarb root is used regulate the digestive tract to treat digestive issues that include diarrhea, constipation, stomach pain, and acid reflux. Rhubarb root softens stool to ease bowel movements and reduces pain from hemorrhoids and tears of the lining of the anus. Rhubarb root is used to treat kidney stones and kidney disease,[89] to chelate heavy metals,[90] to remove acids and mucus, and to **intracellularly cleanse** cells.

Origin: China General commercial dose: One 500 mg capsule General dosage: One capsule two or three times daily

Sage

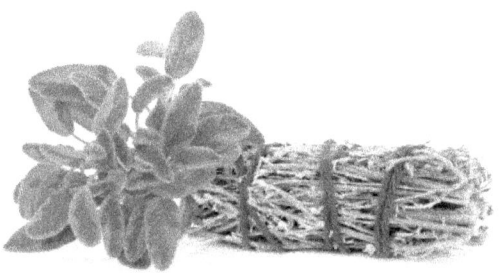

Sage (*Salvia officinalis*) has antioxidant,[91],[92] antimicrobial,[93] anti-inflammatory,[94] antitumor,[95] antidiarrheal,[96] and antiobesity[97] properties. Sage has also been shown to reduce LDL cholesterol and raise HDL cholesterol,[98] improving the HDL/LDL ratio. Sage is used in traditional medicine to improve **memory**,[99],[100] treat **menopausal hot flashes**,[101] reduce gastrointestinal inflammation, nourish the **pancreas**, and treat **diabetes.** [102]

Origin: Mediterranean General commercial dose: One 500 mg capsule General dosage: Two capsules once daily or one capsule twice daily

Santa Maria

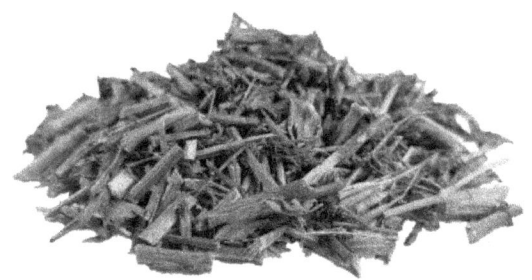

Santa Maria (*Tagetes lucida*, pericón, hierbanis, yerbanís, Mexican marigold, Mexican tarragon) has antifungal and antibacterial,[103] antidepressant,[104] antioxidant and analgesic,[105] and anti-inflammatory[106] properties. Santa Maria is used in traditional medicine to treat diarrhea, abdominal pains, respiratory infections, rheumatism, and inflammatory skin diseases. Santa Maria has **psychoactive** properties and is used to **relax nerves**.

Origin: Central America, Mexico General dose: Santa Maria is usually consumed as an infusion/tea to enhance dreams and visualization—2–4 oz.

standard infusion. Standard infusion: 1 tablespoon herb to 1

cup/8 oz. of boiling water. Steep the herb in the boiling water for 15–20 minutes.

General commercial dose: One 400 mg capsule General dosage: One or two capsules one or two times daily

Sapo

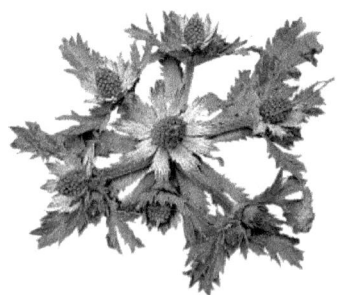

Sapo (*Eryngium carlinae*, yerba del sapo, hierba del sapo, grass frog, grass toad) has hypolipidemic,[107] antioxidant,[108] and anti-inflammatory[109] properties. Sapo is used in traditional medicine to lower cholesterol and triglyceride levels in the blood and arteries. Sapo is used to treat gallstones and **kidney** stones.

Origin: Central America, Mexico General commercial dose: One 400 mg capsule General dosage: Two capsules two or three times daily with meals

Sarsaparilla

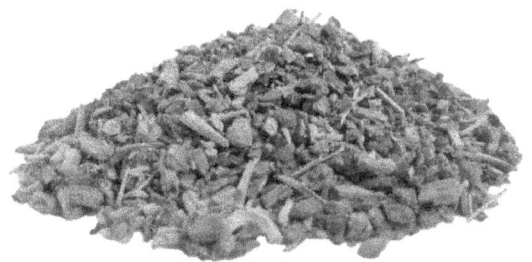

Sarsaparilla (*Smilax, Hemidesmus indicus*) can refer to two species of plant, *Smilax* or *Hemidesmus indicus*. *Smilax* comes from South America, and *Hemidesmus indicus* comes from India, and they have similar properties. They have anti-inflammatory, antiulcer, antioxidant,[110] anticancer,[111] diaphoretic, and diuretic properties. Sarsaparilla has been shown to **bind with toxins** for their removal from the blood and body.[112] Sarsaparilla is used in traditional medicine to treat skin conditions like psoriasis and leprosy, rheumatoid arthritis and joint pain, headaches, colds, and sexual impotence.

Origin: Mexico, Jamaica, India General commercial dose: One 450 mg capsule General dosage: One capsule two times daily

Sea Moss

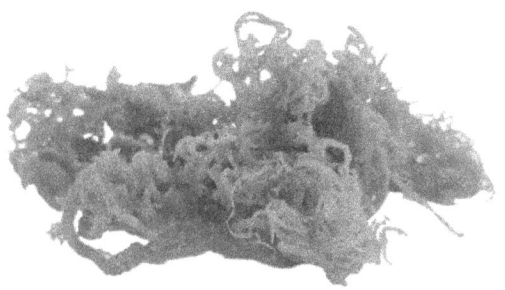

Sea moss (*Chondrus crispus,* Irish moss) has antibacterial,[113],[114] anti-inflammatory,[115] and laxative properties. Sea moss is used for its demulcent properties to sooth irritated mucous membranes from colds, coughs, bronchitis, tuberculosis, gastric ulcers, and intestinal problems. Sea moss is used to support **joint and skin health**, and its wide range of nutrients serve as a natural mineral supplement.

Origin: Atlantic Ocean coastal area General commercial dose: One 400 mg (powder) capsule General dosage: One capsule two times daily (Commercial doses vary greatly, because the properties of sea moss make it more of a natural nutritional supplement rather than a medicinal herb. Sea moss is used in greater quantities to make seamoss beverages and gels.)

Sensitiva

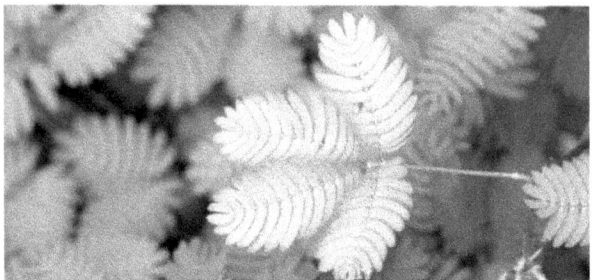

Sensitiva (*Mimosa sensitiva, Mimosa pudica*) has **antidepressant**,[116] anticonvulsant,[117] antibacterial,[118] diuretic, antioxidant,[119] anti-inflammatory,[120] and aphrodisiac properties.[121] Sensitiva is used in traditional medicine to relieve hemorrhoid and arthritis pain, stop bleeding, and treat **uterine infections**. Sensitiva is also used to increase **sexual desire and libido**.

Origin: Central America General commercial dose: One 500 mg capsule General dosage: One capsule two times daily *(Medical caution: sensitiva has shown antifertility properties in laboratory settings using rats. Women who are pregnant are cautioned not to use sensitiva.)*

Shea Butter

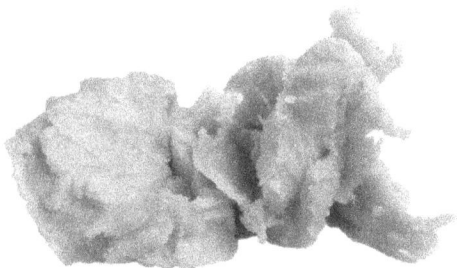

Shea butter (*Vitellaria paradoxa, Butyrospermum paradoxa, Butyrospermum parkii*) is the nut is the shea tree *Vitellaria paradoxa* and is a traditional African plant food. It is popularly used for skin treatment. Shea butter made from the shea nut is rich in skin protective fatty acids, nutrients, and phytonutrients. It is used to moisturize the skin, increase elasticity, and treat conditions like blemishes, wrinkles, sunburn, eczema, and small wounds.

Origin: Africa Application: Shea butter is used as a cream and is applied directly to the skin.

Tila

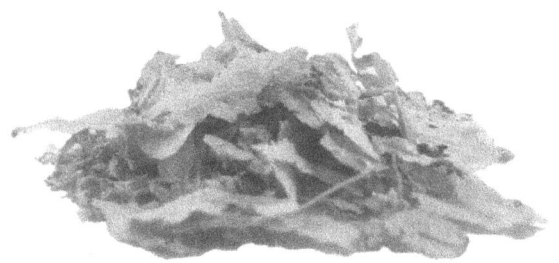

Tila (*Tilia*, linden, basswood) has antioxidant,[122] neuroprotective,[123] anticonvulsant and antiseizure,[124] antispasmodic, anti-inflammatory,[125] anticancer,[126] and diuretic properties. Linden is used in traditional medicine to support the immune system, **relax nerves**, relieve depression, and treat insomnia, fever, headaches, migraines, **inflammatory skin conditions**, and the liver and gallbladder.

Origin: North America, Asia, Europe General commercial dose: One 500 mg capsule General dosage: One capsule two or three times daily

Urtila Oil

Urtila oil (*Urtila dioica, Urtica dioica*, see Nettle) extracted from the nettle plant is used as a hair conditioner and to support oil production in the scalp.

Valerian

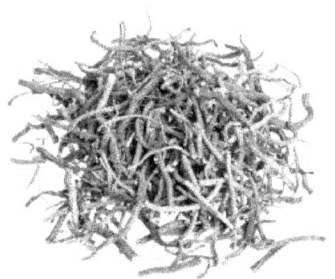

Valerian (*Valerianu officinalis* L Veleriana, valerian, capon's tail, all-heal, garden heliotrope, English valerian, Vermont valeria, setwall, wild valerian) has **sedative**,[127] anticonvulsant,[128] antianxiety, and antidepressant[129] properties. It **relieves anxiety**, nervousness, exhaustion, headache, and hysteria. Valerian is used to relax and **strengthen the uterus**.[130]

Origin: Asia, Europe General commercial dose: One 500 mg capsule General dosage: Two or three capsules before bedtime *(Medical caution: women who are pregnant should consult with a physician.)*

Yellow Dock

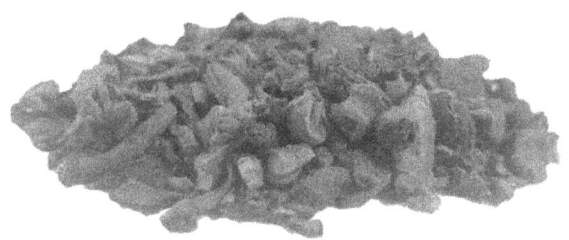

Yellow dock root (*Rumex crispus*, curly dock) has antioxidant,[131] antimicrobial,[132] antibacterial,[133] anti-inflammatory,[134] and analgesic and antipyretic[135] properties. Yellow dock stimulates bile production, aiding in the digestion of fat, and stimulates bowel movement to clear the digestive tract. Yellow dock has been used in traditional medicine as a **blood purifier** and **liver and gallbladder cleanser** and to clean the lymphatic system.

Origin: Africa, Western Asia, Europe General commercial dose: One 500 mg capsule General dosage: Two capsules two times daily *(Medical caution: consult a physician if you have a history of kidney stones.*
)

Yohimbe

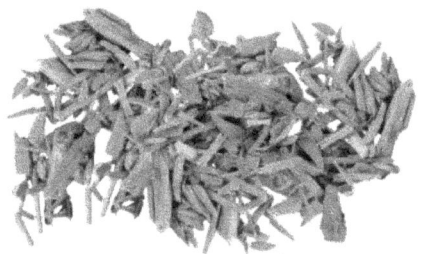

Yohimbe (*Corvanthe yohimbe, Pausinystalia johimbe*, yohimbe bark, yohimbine) has antiobesity,[136],[137] antidepressant,[138] and libido-enhancing[139] properties. Yohimbe is used in traditional medicine to **increase sexual desire** and to reverse erectile impotence. Though yohimbe is used more often for male libido, it is also effective in increasing female sexual desire and performance.

Yohimbe is used as a ground herb made from the bark. Yohimbine is the active ingredient in Yohimbe, and manufacturers extract the yohimbine and sell it as a concentrated extract. It is also made synthetically Yohimbine is not natural and isn't recommended. The ground bark is less potent than the extract, but is safer to use. It takes larger doses of ground yohimbe bark to be as effective as yohimbine. Even so, the natural yohimbine alkaloid in yohimbe is very strong, and it takes very little to support increased libido. If you purchase commercial capsules, make sure the ingredients say yohimbe bark and not extract.

Origin: Western and Central Africa General (bark) commercial dose: One 500 mg (bark) capsule General (bark) dosage: One capsule two to three times daily with water. Its effect builds in the body over time. You may want to start with one capsule daily.

(Medical caution: yohimbe and its yohimbine alkaloid compound are very strong. Do not exceed the recommended dosage. Yohimbe increases heart rate significantly.)

OLD SEBI HERBS

The Dr. Sebi Estro product, which supports the female reproductive system, has been totally redesigned and certain herbs aren't used in the product any more.

Current Estro Product

Damiana (*Tunera diffusa*) Hydrangea (Hortensia) Sarsaparilla (Cocolmeca) Sea moss (*Chondrus crispus*)

Past Estro Product

* Indicates herbs no longer used in the Estro product.

Damiana (*Tunera diffusa*) ***Paeonia** (Peony, paeonia lactiflora, albiflora) ***Senecio** (*Senecio gracilis* liferoot, *Senecio aureus*, false valerian, ragwort, golden senecio) ***Bulgaris** (Vulgaris, mugwort) *** Sempervivum** (Houseleek) ***Pinguicula** (Butterworts) ***Catnip** (*Nepeta Cataria*, catmint, cataria vulgaris) ***Lipoia Tryphylla** (*Lippia triphylla Lipoia citriodora*, Hierbaluisa, lemon verbena)

OTHER-SEBI HERBS

The herbs Dr. Sebi has isolated in his compounds are extensive and address the reversal of disease in numerous and various ways. His compounds have been documented to reverse chronic diseases. Dr. Sebi has spoken about the use and benefits of other herbs that are not necessarily part of the Dr. Sebi cell food compounds, but are used at his USHA village in Honduras.

Guinea Hen Weed

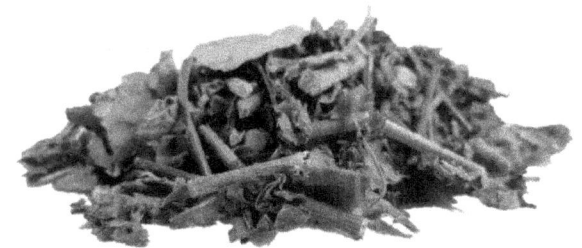

Guinea hen weed (*Petiveria alliacea*, anamu, tipi, apacin, mucura, guine, feuilles ave, herbe aux poules, petevere a odeur ail, mapurite, and gully root) has antimicrobial,[140] **anticancer**,[141] antitumor,[142] antiviral,[143] antioxidant, [144] diuretic, and **anti-HIV**[145] properties. Guinea hen weed is used in traditional medicine to reverse cancer, reduce muscle spasms and fever, relax nerves, relieve pain, lower blood-sugar levels, and treat bacterial, fungal, and virus infections.

Origin: The Caribbean, Central and South America General dose: Guinea hen weed is usually consumed as an infusion/tea. 4 oz. of infusion/decoction of leaves and branches, two to three times daily.

Infusion: 1 tablespoon herb to 8 oz. of boiling water. Steep the herb in the boiling water for 15–20 minutes.

General (capsule) commercial dose: One 500 mg capsule General dosage: One capsule one to two times daily with a meal *(Medical caution: women who are pregnant should avoid anamu, because it can stimulate uterine contractions.)*

Mullein

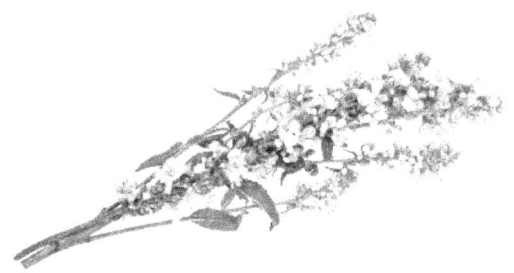

Mullein (*Verbascum, Verbascum thapsus*, Aaron's rod, Indian tobacco, Jacob's staff, Peter's staff, blanket leaf, Bullock's lungwort, cow's lungwort, feltwort, hare's beard, lady's foxglove, mullein leaf) has antiparasitic and antispasmodic,[146] antibacterial,[147] antiviral,[148] anti-inflammatory,[149] antitubercular,[150] and anti-influenza[151] properties. Mullein is used primarily as an expectorant to remove mucus from the respiratory tract, including the lungs.

Origin: Africa, Asia General commercial dose: One 500 mg capsule General dosage: Two capsules two or three times daily

NON-SEBI HERBS

Black seed is a non Sebi herb but I do find value in it. Black seed (*Nigella sativa*) is likely the most scientifically studied herb. It is called the "cure all disease," except for death.

Black Seed

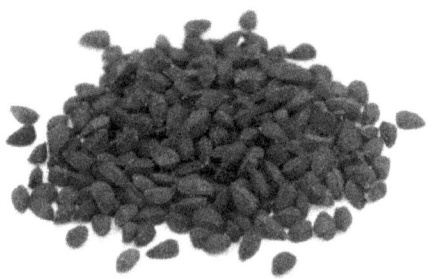

Black seed (*Nigella Sativa*) is commonly referred to as black cumin. *Nigella sativa* is actually a different plant than black cumin. *Nigella sativa* belongs to the Ranunculaceae family, whereas black cumin belongs to the Apiaceae family and is known as *Bunium bulbocastanum*. *Bunium bulbocastanum* is a cousin of cumin and is not related to *Nigella sativa*. Black cumin has different properties from black seed (*Nigella sativa*) and shouldn't be confused with it.

Nigella sativa has analgesic,[152] antimicrobial,[153] antifungal,[154] anti-inflammatory,[155] antioxidant,[156] antiulcer,[157] anticancer,[158],[159] antidiabetic,[160],[161] antiasthmatic,[162] antiepileptic,[163] hepatoprotective (liver protecting),[164] **anti-HIV**,[165] and blood-pressure-regulating[166] properties.

Origin: South and Southwest Asia General commercial dose: One 500 mg capsule General dosage: Two capsules one or two times daily

CHAPTER 5:

HERBAL COMBINATIONS

Specific herbs are used together to address the same condition or area of the body. The doses are reduced in these situations from the doses used for the single herbs. Though herbs can address the same condition or area of the body, they do so in different ways. Cells have receptors that only allow in specific nutrients and phytonutrients. Research has shown that phytonutrients bind to specific receptors of specific cells.[167] Cells in one part of an organ can have different receptors for different nutrients and phytonutrients than another part of the same organ. For example, the phytonutrients in kale are associated with lower risk of colon cancer in the middle and right side of the body, while apples are associated with lower risk of colon cancer in the lower left side of the body.[168]

Unlike pharmaceutical drugs that are made synthetically to mimic one specific phytonutrient in an herb or plant, an herb contains a wide range of phytonutrients that address a wide range of conditions or organs. The nutrients and phytonutrients in an herb work in a synergistic way, compared to a single nutrient or phytonutrient. The variety of nutrients and phytonutrients in an herb and their ability to support multiple functions and organs is also ideal, because no organ or metabolic function truly operates in isolation from the rest of the body.

All functions are interconnected, and the wide variety of nutrients and phytonutrients in one herb helps sustain homeostasis throughout the body. An herb is also concentrated in some nutrients and phytonutrients and less concentrated in others. This means the herb will have a greater healing effect in one or several areas of the body and less of a healing effect in others. Combining herbs to target a specific area of the body will increase the herbs' efficacy in healing and reversing disease in that area of the body.

DR. SEBI'S HERBAL PRODUCTS

The herbalist Dr. Sebi has been instrumental in distinguishing the better alkaline herbs from the hybrid herbs that saturate the market. He has also been a blessing because he put together herbal packages consisting of various herbs in specific doses to address various ailments. He has taken the guesswork out of knowing which are the better alkaline herbs to use and how much to use.

I have covered the properties of many of the herbs Dr. Sebi uses in his herbal packages. You should have a clear understanding of the properties of any traditional or pharmaceutical medicine you put into your body and their effects on the body. Having this understanding also helps promote a positive attitude about the herbs' efficacy, which can increase their efficacy through the power of the mind and its suggestion. This is called the placebo effect, where there is a beneficial effect that is attributed to a person's belief in the treatment.

I was interested in learning herbalism and have studied the properties of herbs and how they are administered. Though herbal medicine is made from natural plants, these herbs are concentrated with phytonutrients and are not normally consumed as food because of their concentration. These phytonutrients have been studied and have been shown to be useful in reversing disease. Around a half of the pharmaceutical drugs used are synthetic versions of the natural phytonutrients. The difference with the pharmaceutical drugs is single phytonutrients are isolated, synthesized, and concentrated, making their use more potent and also more dangerous. The natural amount and ratio of phytonutrients in herbs make their consumption far less problematic, but consuming too much at a time can cause the body to cleanse too quickly, which can overwhelm organs.

Dr. Sebi put together herbal combinations that are safe to consume, support alkalinity, and support the reversal of disease. This is a listing of Dr. Sebi's products. You can find out more about their herbal contents and purchase his herbal packages at **drsebiscellfood.com**.

Cell Products

- Banju
- Bio Ferro
- Bromide Plus
- Estro

- Eva Salve
- Eyewash
- Green Food Plus
- Hair Follicle Fortifier
- Hair food Oil
- Iron Plus
- Testo
- Tooth Powder
- Uterine Wash & Oil
- Viento

Packages

- **All Inclusive Package:** Products Included (20 products): Chelation 1, Chelation 2, Fucus Capsules, Fucus Liquid, L.O.V., Lymphalin, Lupulo, Banju (2), Bio Ferro Tonic (2), Bromide Plus Capsules, Bromide Plus Powder, Bio Ferro Capsules, Green Food, Viento, Iron Plus (2), Endocrine, Testo (for male patients) or Estro (for female patients).
- **Advanced Package:** Products Included (10 products): Chelation 1, Chelation 2, Lymphalin, Fucus Liquid, Lupulo, Bio Ferro Capsules, Bromide Plus Capsules, Viento, Green Food & Iron Plus.
- **Booster Package:** Products Included (7 products): Chelation 2, Lymphalin, Fucus Liquid, Bio Ferro Capsules, Bromide Plus Capsules, Viento & Green Food.
- **Support Package:** Products Included (5 products): Chelation 2, Lymphalin, Bio Ferro Capsules, Bromide Plus Capsules & Viento.
- **Small Cleansing Package:** Chelation2, Bio Ferro and Viento.

It is better to seek the help of a trained herbalist when taking and combining herbs. I am very inquisitive and love to understand how things work. I love herbalism and the healing properties of plants, so I decided to study herbs, their properties, and combining herbs. I have provided information to assist in understanding the efficacy of certain herbs, their dosage, and their application.

COMBINING HERBS

(For educational purposes only. This information has not been evaluated by the Food and Drug Administration. This information is not intended to diagnose, treat, cure, or prevent any disease.) A very important thing to remember is though the herbs I covered are shown to have various healing properties, these herbs work best with the alkaline plant foods on Dr. Sebi's nutritional guide. Taking these herbs while consuming acidic foods like meat, dairy, and processed foods will reduce the efficacy of the herbs in reversing disease. These herbs help alkalize the body and help restore the health of the organs and metabolic processes of the body.

I have put together a list of combinations of herbs based on their properties in addressing specific conditions. **It is very important to drink the recommended one gallon of (spring) water because most of the herbs are diuretics and strip water from the body**. Drinking the recommended amount of water will also dilute toxins moving through the kidneys for excretion, which will take pressure off the kidneys. It is also very important to only eat from the nutritional guide because the foods will saturate the body with nutrients, phytonutrients, and fiber that will help unclog the colon, which is the body's solid-waste-removal system. Some of these herbal combinations may be very similar but not the same as the combinations Dr. Sebi has in his herbal packages.

Parts

I combine a large amount of herbs using a standard part. I then store the herbal mixture in a glass jar with a lid. I encapsulate the herbal mixture in 00 standard capsules containing approximately 500 mg of the herbal mixture.

If I combine five herbs whose individual dose is 500 mg (approximately a quarter teaspoon), and their individual recommended dosage is the same (two or three times a day), I mix one cup of each ground or coarsely ground herb together and add the mixture to a jar. I use a blender to thoroughly mix the herbs together. One cup is the "part" I use. Instead of one cup, I could use a half cup as the part and combine a half cup of each herb.

I could combine five herbs with four of the herbs having an individual dose of 500 mg and one of the herbs having a dose of 250 mg. Using one cup as the "part," I would combine one cup each of the four herbs, and a half cup of the one herb.

The trickiest part is combining herbs that have different dosages. The "dose" is the amount, and the dosage is how many times the dose is used. The dose for one herb could be a 500 mg capsule, and the dosage could be two capsules two or three times daily. The dose for another herb could be a 500 mg capsule, and the dosage could be one capsule two or three times daily. The dosage for the second herb would be half that of the first herb, though the dose is the same. This comes out to be one part of the first herb and a half part of the second herb. Since both herbs are being used for the same condition, it isn't necessary to take the full dosage recommended for each herb. Mix the herbs thoroughly, encapsulate the herbs into 500 mg capsules, and take two capsules two or three times daily.

The following combinations of herbs are based on 500 mg capsules, which is approximately a quarter teaspoon. The "part" to use will depend on amount of mixed herb you want to make. You can use one-half or one cup as the "part" or a larger part depending on how big your container is. I put together the following combination of herbs for educational purposes to give an understanding of how to combine herbs. The herbs may be the same or similar to herbs in Dr. Sebi's compounds, and the ratio of herbs may be different.

(Read the information about each herb to learn about its properties and caution if applicable.)

The Foundation

The "Foundation" is a set of herbs used to clean the liver, kidneys, and blood. These herbs provide a general cleaning to help relieve pressure put on the whole body by the body's nutrient-delivery system (the blood) being compromised by pathogens and toxins. The pathogens and toxins are circulated throughout the body, which compromises the health of the entire body. The blood is also compromised by an unbalanced water-to-electrolyte ratio, which compromises electrical activity in cells throughout the body. Strengthening the **liver** supports its ability to efficiently remove pathogens and toxins from the **blood**, and strengthening the **kidneys** supports their ability to efficiently balance the electrolytes and water in the blood. This combination is similar to the main ingredients in Dr. Sebi's Bio Ferro.

The Foundation is used by itself as a general cleanser or in tandem with other herbal combinations. The more combinations you use together,

the more you will cleanse the entire body down to the intracellular level.

1 part **burdock root**—Blood purifier, liver cleanser, kidney cleanser 1 part **yellow dock**—Blood purifier, liver cleanser, kidney cleanser ½ part **sarsaparilla**—Binds with toxins 1 part **elderberry**—Removes pathogens 1 part **hydrangea root**—Breaks up calcification Mix all parts thoroughly in blender. Make 500 mg capsules or quarter-teaspoon doses.

Dosage: two capsules two or three times daily.

Calcification Remover

Calcification of soft tissue throughout the body obstructs the entry of nutrients and phytonutrients to tissue and cells.

1 part **hydrangea root**—Dissolves kidney stones, cleans lymphatic system ½ part **cascara sagrada**—Breaks up intestinal waste ½ part **red clover**—Breaks up waste in lymphatic system, blood purifier Mix all parts thoroughly in blender. Make 500 mg capsules or quarter-teaspoon doses.

Dosage: two capsules two times daily.

Pancreas and Endocrine Support

This mixture strengthens the pancreas and endocrine system, controls blood-sugar levels, and is used to reverse **diabetes**. Dr. Sebi uses guaco, huereque, nopal, prodijiosa, and contribo in his "Endocrine" compound. I left contribo out of this herbal combination because of its toxicity. Contribo should be administered by an herbalist. I also added sage.

½ part guaco—Removes inflammation, mucus, and candida ½ part huereque—Lowers blood-sugar level 1 part nopal—Reduces type 2 diabetes, high cholesterol, obesity ½ part prodijiosa—Stimulates pancreas secretions, reduces blood sugar level, and induces a vivid dream state 1 part sage—Lowers glucose level Mix all parts thoroughly in blender. Make 500 mg capsules or quarter-teaspoon doses.

Dosage: three capsules two or three times daily.

Gut and Cell Cleanser

The digestive tract is a major area for the proliferation of various diseases. The digestive tract contains beneficial bacteria that serve as a major part (80 percent) of the immune system and protect the body against harmful bacteria, fungus, and other organisms. Cleansing and repairing the cells in the digestive tract and rebalancing the beneficial flora keeps harmful fungus like candida in check. Candida overgrowth is associated with several diseases of the gastrointestinal tract, including inflammatory bowel diseases (IBD) like Crohn's disease (CD) and ulcerative colitis (UC).[169] Candida is also associated with gastric ulcers and **lupus**, and it affects the whole body, resulting in diseases like vaginal yeast infection (candidal vulvovaginitis or vaginal thrush), penis infection (candidal balanitis), and mouth infection (oral candidiasis). These are also areas of herpes outbreaks. These herbs are used to restore the health of the digestive tract, and in doing so, they help to restore the balance of the whole body. This combination can increase bowel movements to three to six times a day.

Dr. Sebi uses cascara sagrada, prodijiosa, and rhubarb root in his chelation 2 product. His chelation 1 contains blessed thistle. I combine the two together.

½ part <u>cascara sagrada</u>—Restores tone and health of intestines by stimulating peristaltic motion to break up and remove putrid waste in diverticula; stimulates stomach, liver, and pancreas secretions ½ part <u>prodijiosa</u>—Stimulates pancreas and liver secretions to aid the digestive process ½ part <u>rhubarb root</u>—Cleanses heavy metals, kills harmful bacteria, addresses digestive issues, cleans and strengthens the digestive tract 1 part <u>blessed thistle</u>—Kills fungus, stimulates the upper digestive tract, increases circulation and oxygen delivery to the brain to support brain function, and supports heart and lung function Mix all parts thoroughly in blender. Make 500 mg capsules or quarter-teaspoon doses.

Dosage: two or three capsules two times daily.

Brain and Nerve Support

This combination relaxes nerves and muscles. It is used to address brain and nerve issues including attention deficit disorder (ADD) and attention deficit hyperactivity disorder (ADHD). Dr. Sebi's "Banju" product contains Santa Maria, blue vervain, burdock root, and elderberry. The "Foundation" contains burdock root and elderberry, and it works well with "Brain and Nerve Support" in calming and supporting the health of the brain and nerves.

1 part <u>Santa Maria</u>—Nerve and muscle relaxant, antidepressant 1 part <u>blue vervain</u>—Heals nerve damage, antianxiety 1 part <u>tila</u>—Relieves headaches, migraines, inflammation, and depression; relaxes nerves; anticonvulsant 1 part <u>lavender</u>—Relieves migraines, body pain, and nerve issues; anticonvulsant Mix all parts thoroughly in blender. Make 500 mg capsules or quarter-teaspoon doses.

Dosage: two or three capsules two times daily.

Uterine Support (Antifibroid)

This combination nourishes the female endocrine system and supports estrogen balance. Hormonal imbalance is a primary reason for the development of fibroids.

1 part <u>damiana</u>—Balances hormones to shrink fibroids 1 part <u>hydrangea</u>—Anti-inflammatory, antiseptic, dissolves calcium deposits in soft tissue 1 part <u>sarsaparilla</u>—Increases sexual desire 1 part <u>sea moss</u>—Supports connective tissue in vagina ½ part <u>bladderwrack</u>— Antiestrogenic effects lower the risk of estrogen-dependent diseases Mix all parts thoroughly in blender. Make 500 mg capsules or quarter-teaspoon doses.

Dosage: two to three capsules two to three times daily.

Vaginal Canal Wash

Use whole pieces of herbs. This combination restores the natural balance of flora in the vaginal canal.

1 part <u>arnica</u> flowers—Antiseptic, reduces inflammation 1 part <u>red clover</u>—Balances estrogen, relieves menopause 1 part <u>hops</u>—Breaks up inflammation 1 part <u>sage</u>—Balances estrogen, relieves menopause Mix all parts together. Use one tablespoon of mixed herbs.
Steep one tablespoon of mixed herbs in one cup of boiled water until the water has cooled to room temperature. Strain the herbs, add the water to a douche bag, and apply to vaginal canal. Use once a month for general maintenance. Use up to three times a week if addressing a vaginal bacterial or fungus condition.

Male Support

Dr. Sebi's Testo product supports male health and contains yohimbe, sarsaparilla, sensitiva, and chaparral. I combine herbs in my male support combination a bit differently.

1 part <u>yohimbe</u> **(bark, not extract)**—Supports libido 1 part <u>damiana</u>—Supports testosterone balance, relaxes anxiety 1 part <u>sensitiva</u>—Aphrodisiac, increases sexual desire 1 part <u>chaparral</u>—Addresses sexually transmitted diseases, cleans cells of penis Mix all parts thoroughly in blender. Make 500 mg capsules or quarter-teaspoon doses.

Dosage: two to three capsules - two times daily.

Cell Energizer

This combination is an iron-rich cell energizer, cleanser, and revitalizer. It delivers iron-and oxygen-rich blood to the brain, nervous system, and **lymphatic system**, and it reduces cravings for additive substances. Cell Energizer is similar to Dr. Sebi's Iron Plus and Viento. The Viento product contains contribo, which I have left out of the combination. Contribo has been found to be harmful to the kidneys if not used properly and should be administered by an herbalist. I used nettle instead of sea moss.

1 part sapo—Anti-inflammatory, supports kidneys, regulates blood sugar ½ part hombre grande—Antifungal, supports immune system and digestive tract ½ part chaparral—Anti-inflammatory, relieves respiratory issues 1 part valerian—Relaxes nerves and supports oxygen delivery to the brain 1 part nettle—General health tonic and blood purifier Mix all parts thoroughly in blender. Make 500 mg capsules or quarter-teaspoon doses.

Dosage: two to three capsules two to three times daily.

Nutrient Support

This is a natural whole-food chlorophyll-rich mineral, vitamin, and phytonutrient supplement. It is similar to Dr. Sebi's Green Food product.

1 part nettle—Joint support, antioxidant, antimicrobial, nutrient support ½ part tila—Antioxidant, nutrient support 1 part nopal—Diabetes, nutrient support ½ part bladderwrack—Iodine, nutrient support 1 part sea moss—Joint and nutrient support Mix all parts thoroughly in blender. Make 500 mg capsules or quarter-teaspoon doses.

Dosage: two or three capsules two to three times daily.

Lupus Buster

Lupus is rooted in candida overgrowth that causes leaky gut. Food, and candida byproducts called mycotoxins, enter the bloodstream and trigger immune and eventually autoimmune reactions. A resulting lupus autoimmune disease attacks the central nervous system, joints, and any part of the body. The following herbal combinations strengthen the digestive tract, remove candida, and strengthen the central nervous system. It is very important to also eat strictly by Dr. Sebi's nutritional guide to reverse lupus.

>   **The Foundation**
>   **Gut and Cell Cleanser**
>   **Brain and Nerve Support**
>   **Cell Energizer**

Complex Diseases

Complex diseases like lupus and cancer are generally linked to an overall breakdown of homeostasis in the body. The root of this breakdown lies in the acidification of the body, which results in the development of chronic disease. Chronic disease manifests as different diseases depending on which area of the body is hit the hardest. All parts of the body are susceptible to chronic disease, including the blood, liver, kidneys, lungs, heart, brain, pancreas, and intestines. ([Please see information on pH in chapter 2.](#)) Unlike Western pharmaceutical practice and medicine, the African Bio Mineral Balance approaches healing as a rebalancing of the whole body through the use of multiple nutrients that effect multiple pathways of an illness. Western medicine, in contrast, uses a single synthetic compound to address one issue or symptom. Symptoms of one complex disease are rooted in the breakdown of various processes in the body. Restoring balance in the body is the key to removing all manifestations of the acidification in the body. This is achieved through consuming alkaline plant foods found on Dr. Sebi's nutritional guide and through cleaning all areas all the body down to the intracellular level using a vast combination of herbs.

>   **The Foundation**
>   **Calcification Remover**
>   **Pancreas and Endocrine Support**
>   **Gut and Cell Cleanser**
>   **Brain and Nerve Support**
>   **Cell Energizer**
>   **Nutrient Support**
>   **Female Support**

www.ingramcontent.com/pod-product-compliance
Lightning Source LLC
Chambersburg PA
CBHW071114030426
42336CB00013BA/2072